Crack  the Vitamin Code

How to Build your Own Supplement Stack. The Secret of Stacking Supplements for Beginners, How to Buy Vitamins and Minerals, and the Benefits of Dietary Supplements.

By Dr. Ernesto Martinez

www.AttaBoyCowboy.com

Also by Dr. Ernesto Martinez

How to Travel the World and Live with No Regrets.
Learn How to Travel for Free, Find Cheap Places to Travel, and Discover Life-Changing Travel Destinations.

How to Boost Your Credit Score Range and Make Money with Credit Cards.
How to Repair Your Credit with Credit Repair Strategies.

How to Become Rich and Successful: Creative Ways to Make Money with a Side Hustle
How to Become a Millionaire: Learn the Best Passive Income Ideas

How to Heal Broken Bones Faster. Bone Fracture Healing Tips. Learn About Bone Fracture Healing Foods, Types of Bone Fractures, and the Five Stages of Bone Healing.

How to Become Rich and Successful. The Secret of Success and the Habits of Successful People.
Entrepreneurship and Developing Entrepreneur Characteristics

How to Lose Weight Without Dieting or Exercise.
Over 250 Ways.
Learn About Foods that Burn Fat, Weight Loss Diets, Weight Loss Tips, Weight Loss Foods, and How to Lose Belly Fat

Cracking the Vitamin Code
How to Build your Own Supplement Stack. The Secret of Stacking Supplements for Beginners, How to Buy Vitamins and Minerals, and the Benefits of Dietary Supplements.

The Hardcore Program
How to build world-class habits and routines. Proven strategies for weight loss, success, and optimal health. How to form yourself into a new you through ritual and routine optimization.

The contents of this book may not be reproduced, duplicated, or transmitted without direct written permission from the author.

Under no circumstances will any legal responsibility or blame be held against the publisher for any reparation, damages, or monetary loss due to the information, either directly or indirectly.

Cracking the Vitamin Code

How to Build your Own Supplement Stack. The Secret of Stacking Supplements for Beginners, How to Buy Vitamins and Minerals, and the Benefits of Dietary Supplements.

© **Copyright 2022** - Ernesto Martinez, eBook, and paperback. All rights reserved.

Legal Notice:
This book is copyright protected. This is only for personal use. You cannot amend, distribute, sell, use, quote or paraphrase any part of the content within this book without the consent of the author.

Disclaimer Notice:
Please note the information contained within this document is for educational and entertainment purposes only. Every attempt has been made to provide accurate, up-to-date and reliable complete information. No warranties of any kind are expressed or implied. Readers acknowledge that the author is not engaging in the rendering of legal, financial, medical, or professional advice. The content of this book has been derived from various sources.

Copyright © 2022 Dr. Ernesto Martinez
All rights reserved.
ISBN: 978-1-64635-032-2 eBook,
978-1-64635-031-5 Paperback, 978-1-64635-103-9 Hardback

Table of Contents

Dedication 1
Introduction 2
The History of Supplements 9
    1. What are Supplements? 12
    2. Why do we need supplements? 13
    3. What's the solution to overconsumption of processed food and depleted farmland? 18
    5. Do supplements work? 22
    6. Some supplements that can cause health risks include: 25
    7. Dietary Supplement Labels 26
    8. Relationship between Nutrition and Disease 27
    9. Nutritional Approach to Health 27
    10. As the World Ages the Need for Supplements Increases. 28
    11. What are Vitamins? 28
    12. Can I get my vitamins from my diet? 31
    13. How are Vitamins and Supplements Made? 36
    14. How to Differentiate Between Herbal Products? 36
    15. What is the Difference Between Concentrated and Standardized Extracts? 40
    16. How are Dietary Supplements Tested? 41
    17. How to Spot Fraudulent Products? 43
    18. How to avoid supplement Scams? 44
    19. Which Supplements are most effective? 46
    20. Does it Matter what Brand of Supplements you Buy? 46

21. Can I take expired Supplements? 48

22. Can I Cut Supplements in Half if I have difficulty swallowing them? 48

23. What are good Resources for Picking Supplements? 48

24. What Vitamin Combinations Should You Avoid? 50

25. Do vitamins and minerals make up for a poor diet? 54

26. Who needs to take supplements? 54

27. How are vitamins and supplements regulated? ..55

28. What to consider when choosing supplements? 56

29. How can I evaluate the quality of a supplement? 56

30. What supplements should I consider? 56

31. How long do supplements stay in my system? ...59

32. How long should I take a supplement before deciding if it works or not? 59

33. Is it OK to take a supplement one day but not the next? 59

34. What is the best supplement form? 59

35. What is the Best Supplement Form? 63

36. What's the difference between the RDA, DRI, and DV for a vitamin or mineral? 63

37. How much should I be taking? 63

38. Can I be healthy without taking supplements? ..64

39. Are probiotics something I should take long-term or only immediately after taking an antibiotic? 65

40. Can supplements interact with prescribed medications? 65

41. Can I trust the health claims made on a supplement box?..65

42. Should I buy synthetic or organic supplements?..66

43. Does taking vitamins make you gain weight?.....66

44. Which vitamins are best taken together?...............68

45. Which vitamins should not be taken together?..68

46. Should I take supplements with food?....................69

47. Five factors that can Interfere with Nutrient Absorption 70

48. Why do multivitamins have vitamins and minerals that counteract? Are multivitamins good?........71

49. What Time of Day Should I Take My Supplements?...73

50. What would a sample vitamin schedule look like? 73

51. Can supplements be used to treat disease?.........74

52. What are probiotics and prebiotics?......................74

53. How do you know if you're taking the right supplements?...75

54. What is chelation?...82

55. Where should I store my supplements?................82

56. How to get started with supplements?..................83

57. Which supplements should you keep, and which ones should you cut out if you need to save money?.....84

58. What type of doctor should I see to have my blood tested? 85

59. What supplements does Dr. Martinez most often recommend to patients?..86

60. What supplements does Dr. Martinez take?.........87

61. How much is too much?...97

62. What are the best Supplements for each category? 102

63. What are the top 5 Supplement Websites?..........110

64. What are the top Supplement Brands?..................110

65. Do I need to take protein powder as part of my supplement program? 112

66. Most commonly used supplements. 113

About the Author...253

Bonus...256

Dedication

Friends are the family we choose, and the bond between friends is beyond the mortal world. Thank you, Michelle, for always being kind, caring, taking the time to listen to a friend, giving heartfelt advice, and for all the service you provided to thousands of patients. I love you, your friend always, Ernesto Martinez.

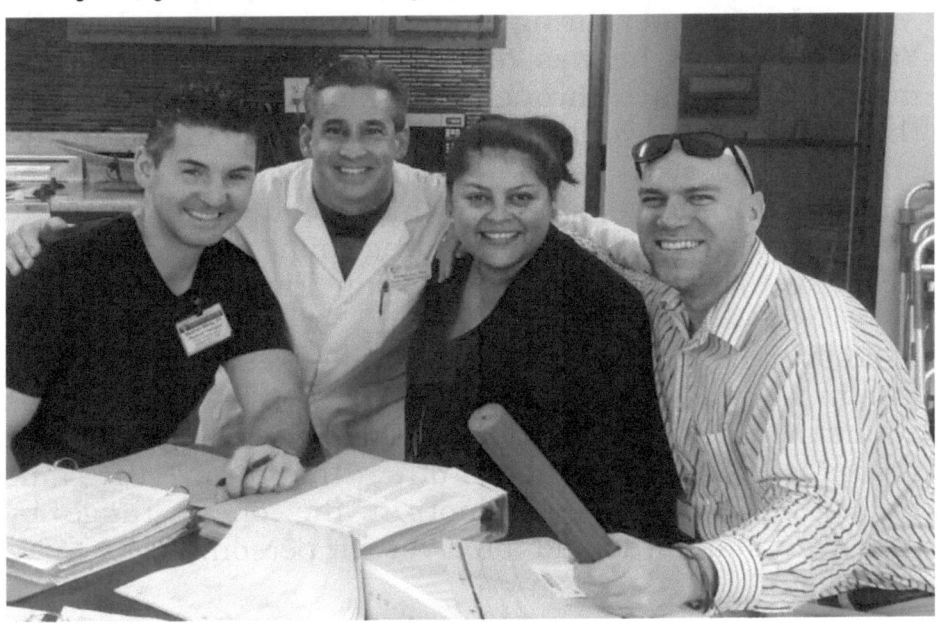

Introduction

It was 2010, and it was my first time in the Southeast Asian country of Myanmar (formerly known as Burma). The land was beautiful, and the archaeological sites were among the best globally. However, I could not overlook how thin the people looked. At 6'2", 210 lb., I could fit two men and a woman inside my body. These were the skinniest people I had ever seen on the planet (I would later see thinner people in North Korea). I remember hiring a rickshaw driver while I was in Yangon, and as he was tugging me around, I could see many of his bones through his skin. I recalled thinking this gentleman would be a perfect specimen for an anatomy class. I could see his bones and muscles perfectly through his skin, which made me decide to switch roles with him and drag him around on the rickshaw. He thought I was being kind. I thought to myself, "I want a body like him." As the young man maneuvered to get into the rickshaw, I remember looking at him sideways and thinking, this guy is so skinny he is about the thickness of a door. If three guys like him stood and pressed up against each other, they'd have the same thickness as me. I was not in the obese range by American standards and am a very fit person.

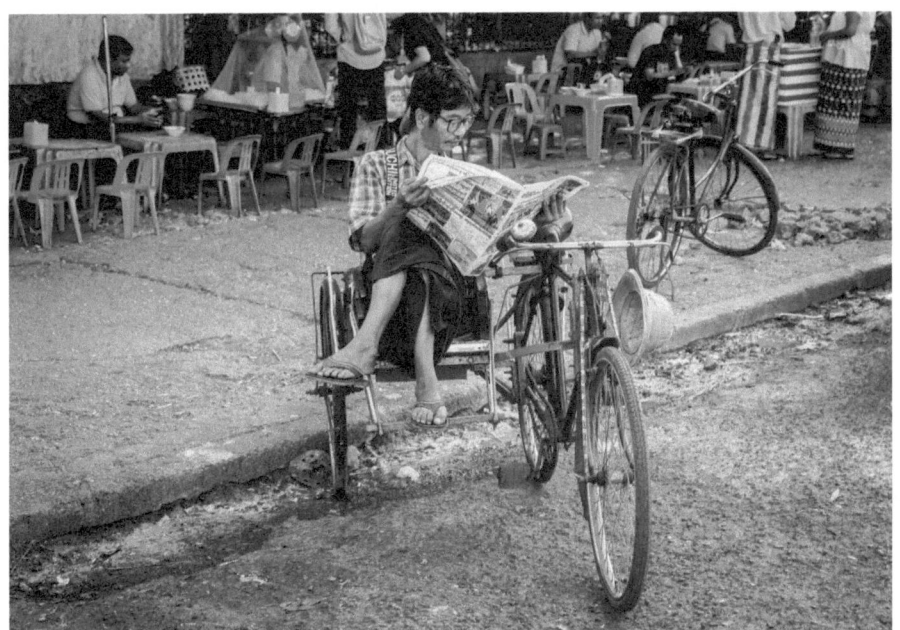

I spent the day with my charming Rickshaw driver. Throughout our conversations, I inquired about his eating habits and access to food. I was trying to figure out why he was so thin. From what he told me, he had sufficient food and could get the sustenance he needed daily for himself and his family. What I did notice was signs of vitamin deficiencies due to malnutrition. He had a very large adam's apple, which sometimes indicates goiter, a disorder caused by iodine deficiency, brittle nails indicative of iron deficiency, and dehydrated skin due to lack of vitamin A.

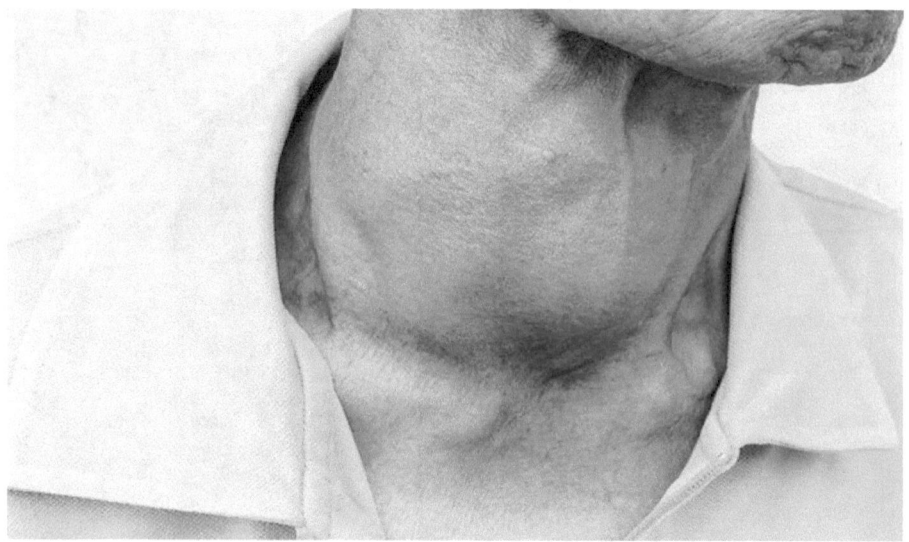

(Goiter caused by iodine deficiency rises as people erroneously switch from plain iodized salt to higher-end salts such as sea salt or pink salt. Salt is salt, and the least expensive iodized table salt is the best for you because it is enriched with iodine. Other salts don't have enough iodine to meet your needs.)

I started researching and discovered that Myanmar (Burma) is among 20 countries where 80% of the children are malnourished. Children who are malnourished between conception and age two are at high risk for impaired physical and mental development, adversely affecting the country's productivity and growth. The three most common micronutrient deficiencies in Myanmar are iodine, iron, and vitamin A. These three micronutrient deficiencies cost the nation about 2.4% of its GDP. Persistent micronutrient deficiencies among children have hampered Myanmar's economic growth and lowered its GDP. In other words, not eating well has long-term social and economic effects on countries.

I assumed the USA would not have these issues, since most people I see are heavy and we are the land of the all-you-can-eat buffets. However, when I compared Myanmar to the USA, I was surprised to find that Americans have even more vitamin deficiency on average due to poor diet and physical inactivity.

According to studies by the National Institute of Health (NIH) and the Centers for Disease Control (CDC), Americans are deficient in not four, but ten nutrients including essential fatty acids, iron, iodine, vitamin C, vitamin D, vitamin B12, folic acid, calcium, vitamin A, and magnesium depending on the population surveyed. These deficiencies cause chronic diseases, such as type 2 diabetes mellitus, cardiovascular disease, cancer, and osteoporosis. Approximately one-half of American adults have at least one preventable chronic disease, and obesity is a significant public health problem in the US, with more than one-third of adults and 17% of children and adolescents classified as obese.

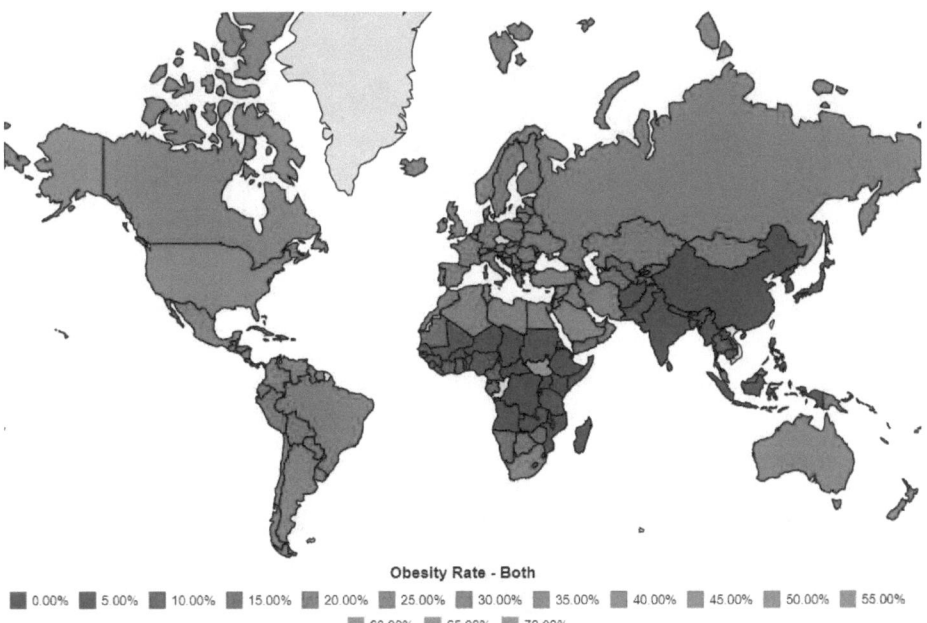

The United States is blessed with an abundance of food, contrasting the great food disparity amongst developed and developing countries. However, unlike the old cliche, more is not always better. Although we have lots of food, we're eating an energy-rich and nutrient-poor diet. While my Burmese friend is eating fresh-picked and home cooked food, he's eating a limited variety of foods that does not support his nutritional needs and his food is being grown on over-farmed soils that lack nutrients, and the farmers lack the economic resources to buy fertilizers to compensate for it.

Inversely the USA has plenty of soil additives and a great variety of fresh foods. Our issue is we degrade the food and remove most of its nutrients by processing and consequently denaturing our food into Franken foods.

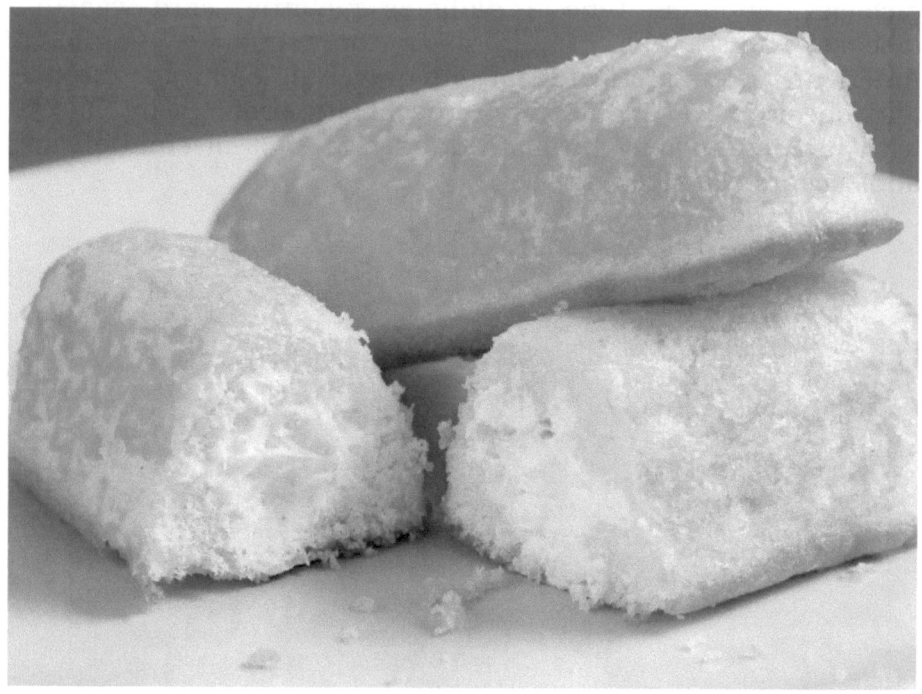

For example, a Twinkie contains 37 ingredients, but only 5 of them are 'recognizable.' Flour, egg, water, sugar, and salt. It also has five types of sugar, and fourteen of the top twenty chemicals made in the U.S.

Heavily processed foods often include unhealthy added sugar, sodium, and fat levels. These ingredients make the food we eat taste better and addictive, which leads to multiple health problems, including obesity, heart disease, high blood pressure, and diabetes. Seventy percent of our calories now come from processed food. Meaning 70% of our food has lost around 90% of its nutrients during processing. The more "modern" or advanced the economy, the more processed foods available to help compensate for the lack of time people have for preparing or eating their food. It's cheaper and faster to eat a "Pop Tart" for breakfast than to prepare a veggie omelet. Every morning, I'm reminded of this when I see 20-30 cars lined up outside McDonald's or Dunkin Donuts waiting to buy high-calorie, low nutrient processed foods to help save time to boost productivity.

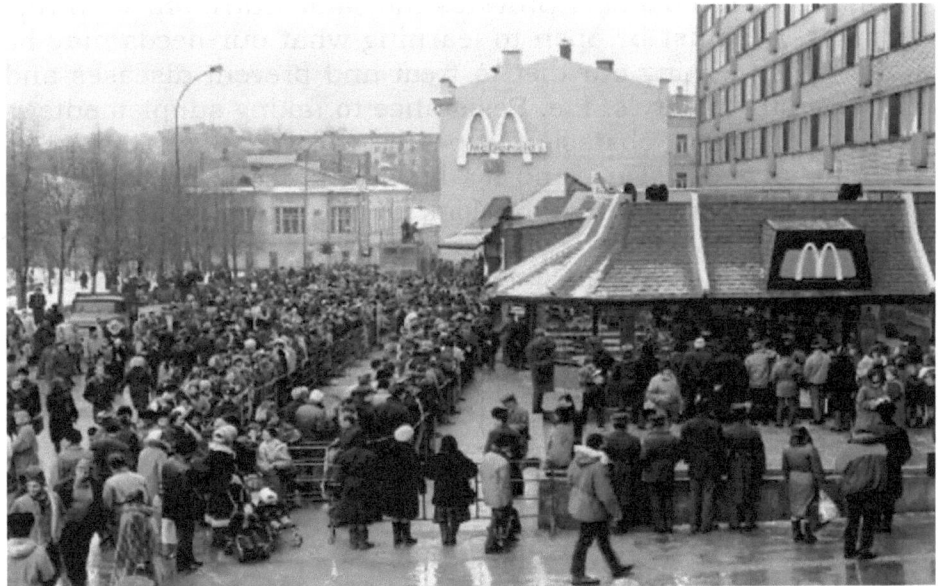

People lined up outside the first McDonald's opening in Russia.

People are sacrificing the quality of their nutrition to dedicate more time to work to buy more material things. In most of the world, it's now much harder to find whole food versus processed foods. The future of human nutrition will include nutritional supplementation as a necessity rather than a supplement to compensate for this trend.

Another issue for people worldwide is not eating a suitable variety of foods. In developed countries, food is mainly processed and does not meet people's daily nutritional requirements. In contrast, developing countries tend to have access to fresher, less processed foods, but less of them and less variety. In addition, due to over farming, the nutrient density of the foods produced is historically lower worldwide due to soil nutrient depletion.

One of the best solutions available is supplementation. Whereas some may question the integrity of taking supplements, I have experienced first-hand with thousands of patients the benefits of supplementation filling the void left by our industrial food supply.

The first step is recognizing that the Earth is changing and Mother Nature no longer provides the same nutrition. With this in mind, we must be open to learning what our needs may be and supplementing our diet to treat and prevent diseases and improve our quality of life. Resistance to taking supplements is often the biggest obstacle for people to overcome. Change is difficult for most of us, and it's hard to accept why you might need supplements when you look in the mirror and look the same as you looked a few days or weeks ago. The benefits of good nutrition can take years before you see the external benefits, even if felt within hours.

For most of us trying to figure out what supplements to take is enough to cause paralysis by analysis and cause some of us to avoid them altogether in fear that we might take the wrong ones, waste our money, or simply poison ourselves. These are the exact concerns I hear from the patients I have the pleasure to serve. Supplement information can be tricky where one day experts fully support a specific health claim, and a month later, public opinion has shifted to support another claim due to a new scientific breakthrough.

The frontiers of science are expanding daily, and we must remain open to further information even when it goes against what we may have believed to be true in the past. As we have learned throughout the Covid-19 pandemic, reality is not static, it changes according to the latest scientific findings. As Charles Darwin said, it's not the smartest or the strongest that survives; it is the most flexible. In terms of your nutrition, the more willing you are to change your dietary habits and supplementation, the less disease you will experience and the greater quality of life you will enjoy.

Keep in mind that specks of nutrients, the size of grains of salt, can be the difference between long-term disability and optimal human performance. This book will give you the tools and the information you need to chart your course in the nutrition supplementation world to help you reach your peak performance and stave off illness.

The History of Supplements

Kazimierz Funk, also known as Casimir Funk, was a Polish and American biochemist, who was among the first to coin the concept of vitamins, which he called "vital amines" or "vitamines." Nutritional research has significantly shortened the period of humans suffering from vitamin deficiencies. The significant discoveries began in the early nineteenth century and ended in the mid-twentieth century. These discoveries helped us understand many health issues. The contributions of epidemiologists, physicians, physiologists, and chemists helped us figure out the role of vitamins in human health. Before these discoveries, deficiencies in proteins, carbohydrates, fats, and minerals were considered the cause of most health problems. With the discovery of vitamins, clinicians figured out that diseases such as rickets, scurvy, beriberi, pellagra, and xerophthalmia were caused by vitamin deficiencies rather than infections or toxins.

As a kid, my favorite disease to read about was Scurvy. It was the most common disease among sailors and pirates during the fifteenth and sixteenth century, particularly when taking long transatlantic journeys during the Age of Discovery. Scurvy is caused by a lack of vitamin C thanks to limited supplies of fruits and vegetables while at sea for long periods. Pirates suffering from scurvy would feel weak and develop spots and lesions on their skin, weak gums, and nose bleeds. The most common places for pirates to find scurvy spots would be on the legs and thighs. The latter stages of the disease saw pirates lose their teeth, suffer from jaundice and open wounds, then eventually die. Aside from the cool name, most kids love to read about pirates. So the word "scurvy" comes to mind every time I see one of the Pirates of the Caribbean movies.

SCURVY

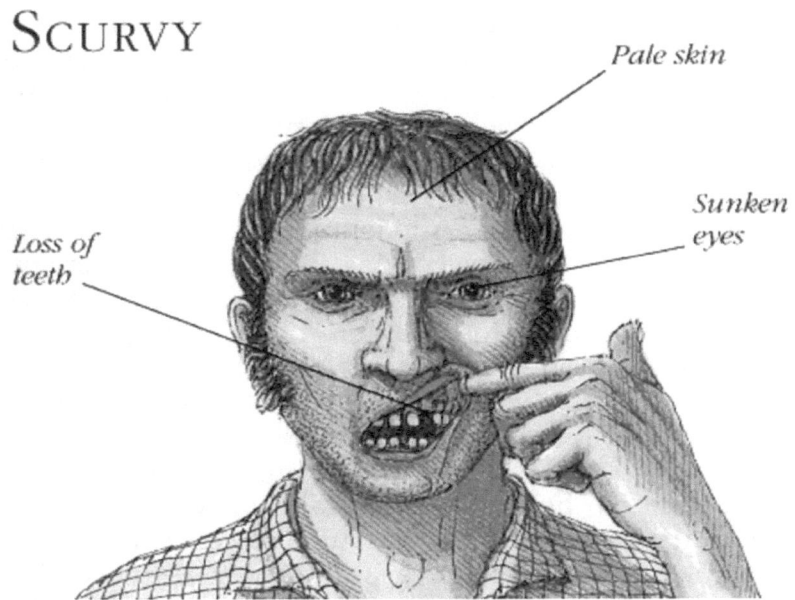

Ultimately, chemists isolated the various vitamins, deduced their chemical structure, and developed vitamin synthesis methods. Our understanding of the vitamins continues to evolve from the initial discovery period. By 2026, the dietary supplement market will grow to 349 billion USD.

After synthesizing and isolating the different types of vitamins our body needs to survive, clinicians started using vitamin supplements to address health issues, and the multivitamin arose from these efforts. Supplements became more popular as agriculture industrialized, resulting in less nutritious foods and processed foods becoming common and leading to a dramatic change in people's diets, including a lack of nutrients. More people started using dietary supplements to make up for changes in society. As a result diseases such as scurvy are now something you mostly read about in books.

Then in 1994, the Dietary Supplement Health and Education Act (DSHEA) was passed as a statute of United States Federal legislation that defines and regulates dietary supplements. Officially defining nutritional supplements as "a product (other than tobacco) intended to supplement the diet that contains one or more of the following dietary ingredients: a mineral; a vitamin; amino acid; an herb or botanical; a dietary substance for use by man to supplement the diet by increasing the total dietary intake; or a concentrate, constituent, metabolite, extract, or combination of any ingredient described." Under the act, supplements are regulated by the FDA for Good Manufacturing Practices under 21 CFR Part 111.

Under DSHEA, dietary supplements are considered food, except for purposes of the drug definition. In addition, a dietary supplement must be labeled as a dietary supplement and intended for ingestion. It must not be represented for use as a conventional food or as a sole item of a meal or the diet. In addition, a dietary supplement cannot be approved or authorized for investigation as a new drug, antibiotic, or biologic unless it was marketed as a food or a dietary supplement before such approval or authorization.

The definition helped differentiate between supplements and the other substances we consume for nutritional benefits. For example, garlic pills are a supplement because they are concentrated with minerals and antioxidants, making them a favored option for people who want the nutritional boost in measured doses without the odor. Because of the concentration, only a limited amount of garlic pills should be consumed at one time. On the other hand, garlic does not fall under the same category, as it is less concentrated. So there's no harm in eating as much as you like.

Another huge difference is that the FDA is not authorized to review the safety and effectiveness of supplements before they're sold; as a result, companies are responsible for testing their products before selling them. Manufacturers who want to use new ingredients must submit a new dietary ingredient (NDI) application with the FDA that explains the information used to determine that the ingredient is safe under recommended use conditions. Because supplements have very little regulation compared to pharmaceutical drugs, it's like the wild wild west for supplement sales, which has caused them to explode in popularity due to the high-profit margins and lack of the expensive rules and research required for pharmaceuticals.

As supplements have become intertwined with the wellness industry, cultural norms change. More people take a holistic view of nutrition, exercise science, and human behavior to come together to form an individual's optimum fitness level. Meanwhile, supplements have become a tool used by fitness professionals to address individual needs.

Due to the availability of health information online, these products are growing in popularity. As more people become knowledgeable and proactive in their wellbeing, we will see many more transformations to our diets and habits.

1. What are Supplements?

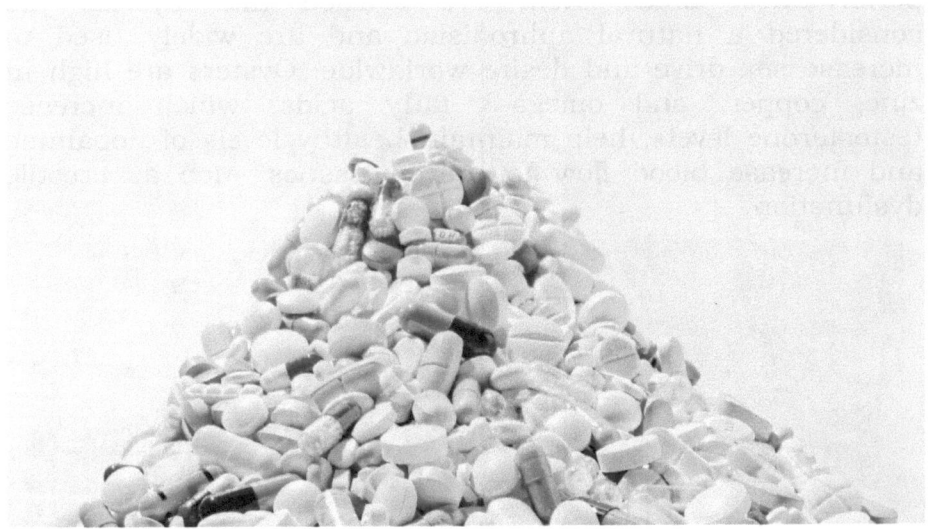

A supplement is just as it sounds, something to be taken in addition to your food. A vitamin is a naturally occurring substance primarily found in food. Supplements are not food and are produced in a laboratory. The Dietary Supplement Health and Education Act (DSHEA) of 1995 classified dietary supplements as ingested through the mouth, whether as a pill, tablet, capsule, soft gel, chewy gummy, chewable tablet, melt-away, powder, drink, or bar.

In fact, the supplements you see in stores are called "synthetic nutrients." They're made in a lab instead of the natural nutrients found in the foods you eat. Supplements range from water-soluble vitamins (which dissolve in water) to herbal supplements, fat-soluble vitamins (stored in the body's fatty tissue and liver), and protein supplements. Supplements are made in various forms, including; pills, powders, liquids, capsules, tablets, and even intravenous supplementation.

When I was 21 years old, I went backpacking and hitchhiking through Mexico for three months. One night while dancing at a nightclub, I noticed that the Mexican guys started ordering rounds of oysters around closing time. The thought was that eating oysters would help them perform in the sack with their girlfriends later that night. Oysters were my first experience with supplements and people's drive to boost performance. Since then, I've learned that oysters are considered a natural aphrodisiac and are widely used to increase sex drive and desire worldwide. Oysters are high in zinc, copper, and omega-3 fatty acids, which increase testosterone levels, help maintain healthy levels of dopamine and increase blood flow to prevent issues such as erectile dysfunction.

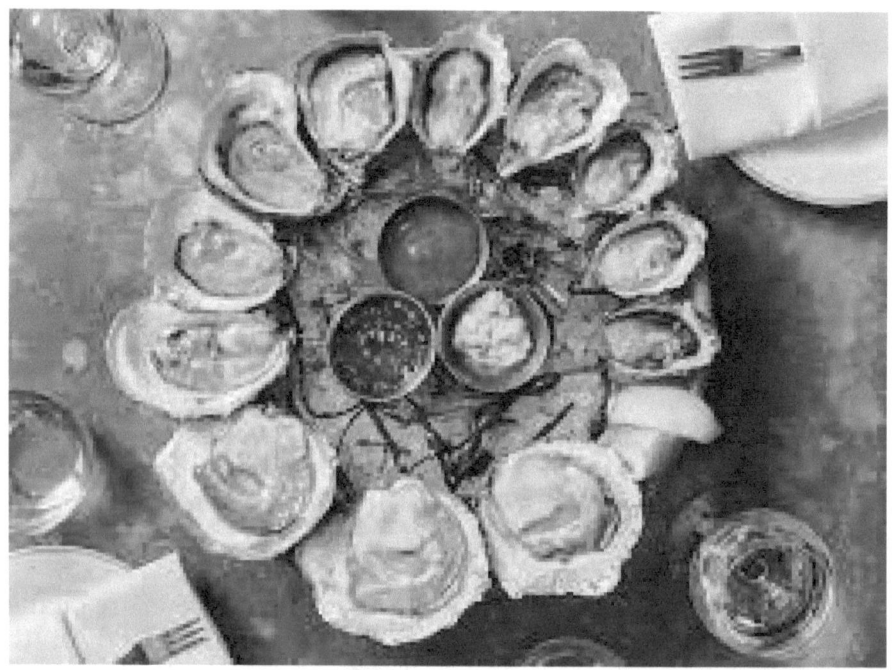

2. Why do we need supplements?

Why couldn't the polar bear take his vitamins? Because the seal was broken.

Due to higher profit margins, processed and fast foods have replaced fresh, nutrient-rich foods as staples in the American diet. Healthy meals are time-consuming and expensive, making them a luxury rather than the standard at dinner tables, and the same trend is happening worldwide.

Research dating back as far as 1936 has shown that the soil of farmland all across the Earth is deficient in micronutrients, lowering nutrient density in produce.

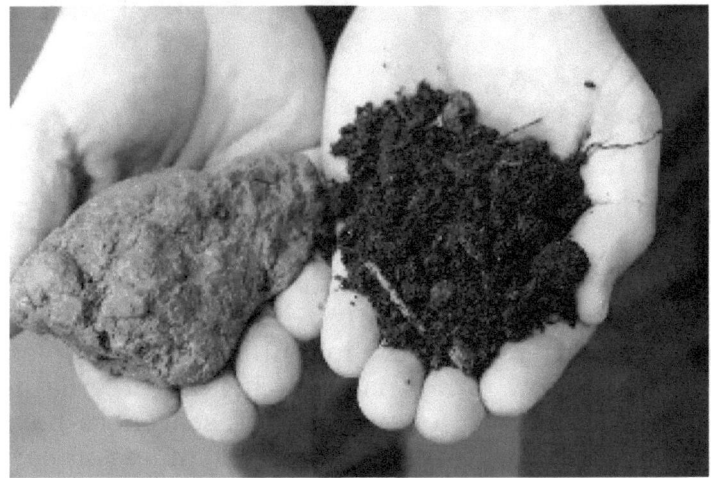

The soil on the left has been treated with chemicals that kill earthworms. The dirt on the right has not been treated with chemicals and is full of worms, insects, and plant matter.

Dirt is amongst the planet's most complex and biodiverse ecosystems, containing nearly a quarter of all species. A cup of soil contains about 10 to 100 million living organisms.

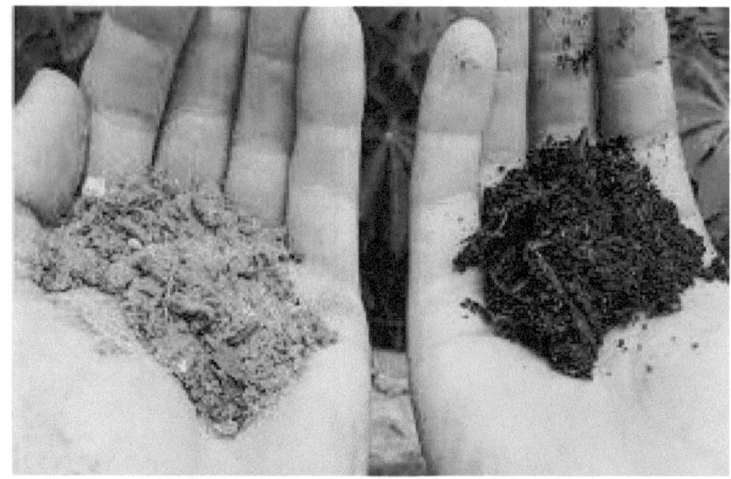

Chemical fertilizers, inorganic fertilizers, and pesticides decrease the quality of the crops and soil fertility. Leading to a decrease in soil quality and poor quality of produce.

Worms provide essential ecosystem benefits like decomposing dead plants, cycling nutrients that plants and animals need to grow to nourish new life, and regulating pests and diseases. In an acre of good soil, researchers have found more than 1 million worms and 1,200 miles of earthworm holes or tunnels.

The greyish color of the soil treated with pesticides is due to microbiological degradation. Bacteria, viruses, fungi, algae, worms, and protozoa live in the upper one foot of soil. Combined, they help keep the soil fertile, and provide a structure, so the most nutrient-dense topsoil is not washed away during irrigation or rain. The topsoil has warmer temperatures, moisture, and organic matter so that microorganisms can thrive and do most of their work, churning the soil and adding nutrients from their waste. Microorganisms are most active in soils with high organic matter, which helps retain moisture in the dirt for plants to grow in and feed the microorganisms.

Dirt like the one pictured to the left treated with pesticides will experience a die-off of microorganisms, typically feed fungus that grows like a web in soil throughout the entire planet and helps hold dirt together. As this fungus dies off, it becomes easier for the more nutrient-dense topsoil to be washed away during irrigation or rain, leaving behind clay-like soil that has a more challenging time retaining moisture, causing less biodiversity, and decreased nutrients for plants and animals. This leads to fewer nutrients and less water in the soil hence its grey color and clay-like appearance compared to the darker (due to increased moisture retention), fluffier (due to burrows by worms) healthy soil that makes it easier for plants to grow on.

In 2003, Canadian researchers compared the current vegetable nutrient content to their content from 50 years ago. The research demonstrated that the mineral content of cabbage, lettuce, spinach, and tomatoes had decreased from 400 milligrams to less than 50 milligrams per serving in the twentieth century. This trend is expected to continue due to overpopulation and over farming to keep up with population growth. The earth is just not being given enough time to replenish itself, so the soil is rapidly being depleted of nutrients, decreasing the nutrient density of produce. According to the U.S. Department of Agriculture (USDA) and the Centers for Disease Control (CDC):

7 out of 10 are deficient in calcium
8 out of 10 are deficient in vitamin E
9 out of 10 Americans are low in potassium
50 % of Americans are deficient in vitamin A, C, & magnesium
Over 50 % of the general population is vitamin D deficient
70 % of elderly Americans are vitamin D deficient
90 % of Americans of color are vitamin D deficient

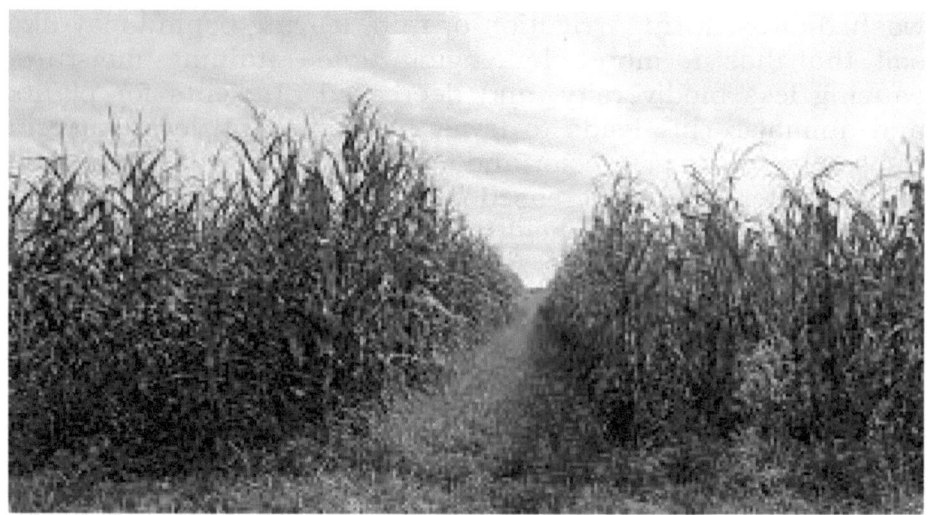

(Corn on the left side is organic versus non-organic corn on the right side, burned by the various chemicals meant to help it grow.)

Iowa is a farming state, and every time I've visited my family there, I got an education about agriculture from the experts. My cousin Rollin worked for the agricultural department, monitoring artificial chemical levels in the soil around the corn crops. He explained how the use of pesticides, herbicides, and fungicides needed to be balanced. Too little would not be effective in growing food, but too much, and you would damage the ecosystem on the farm and surrounding areas for years. Our days started early and consisted of driving our Ford F-150 all over the county, taking soil samples on farms to check chemical levels, and ensuring that people were not using too many synthetic chemicals and polluting the surrounding environment.

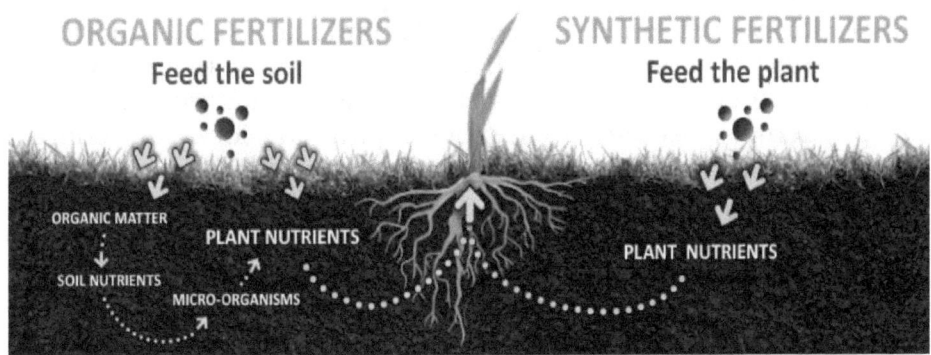

Organic chemicals work to feed the microorganisms in the soil and build up the ecosystem within the ground to produce nutrients that the plants can use and promote a symbiotic relationship. In contrast, artificial chemicals were like a shot of adrenaline; they did nothing for the dirt and went directly into the plant. The problem is that the benefits were short-lived, and they offered a limited scope of advantages compared to the many benefits that organic chemicals created. One of them is around 40% or more nutritious food than food grown with artificial chemicals.

3. What's the solution to overconsumption of processed food and depleted farmland?

Why did the divorced dad have a vitamin D deficiency? He wasn't getting enough Son

For decades, researchers have disputed the necessity of supplements in the diet. However, many now agree supplementation is necessary. Even the American Medical Association recommends all adults take at least a properly dosed multivitamin a day.

Quality supplements can help restore and maintain optimal micronutrient levels. Whether you are a couch potato or an athlete, your diet should be supplemented to reach your health goals.

Increased Use of Supplements

My friend asked me what B vitamins I was taking? I told him it's complex!

According to the Council for Responsible Nutrition's (CRN) consumer survey on dietary supplements in 2020, Americans report their highest overall dietary supplement usage to date, with 77 percent of Americans saying they consume nutritional supplements. People are experiencing a loss of energy, cognitive deficits, and weight gain even though they try to eat healthier and healthier. Many people feel helpless to stop the weight gain and rapid aging of their bodies. In the quest to stop this process, many are looking for alternatives. The survey indicates that most males and females, aged 18+, have continually increased their use of dietary supplements. Adults ages 35 – 54 have the highest use of nutritional supplements at 81 percent. Coincidentally, this is when middle age kicks in and most people start to feel the effects of aging. I can personally attest to that.

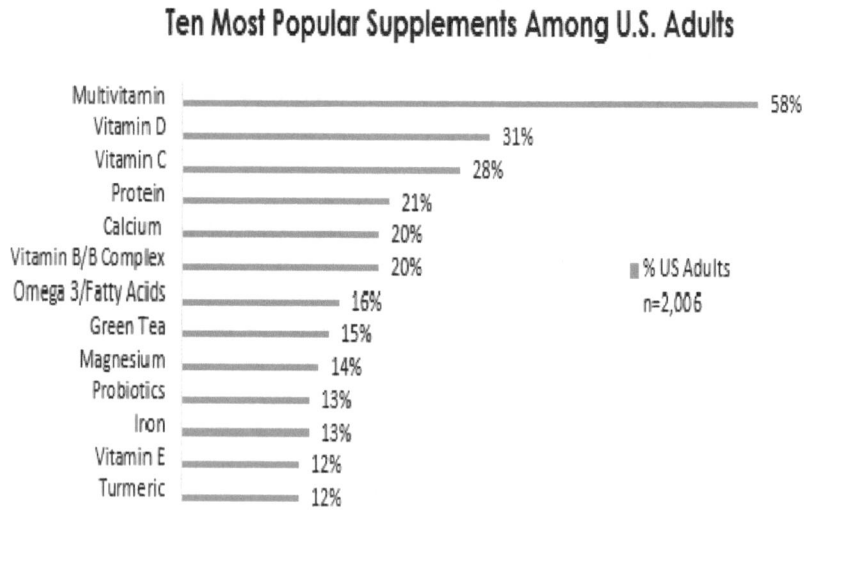

(According to the consumer survey performed by the Council for Responsible Nutrition in 2019, these were the most popular supplements (www.ncbi.nlm.nih.gov).)

Supplement Statistics
77 percent of U.S. adults take dietary supplements.

The following is a breakdown of those 77 percent:
79 percent are female adults
74 percent are male adults
70 percent are adults 18 – 34
81 percent are adults 35 – 54
79 percent are adults are 55+
83 percent are adults with children under 18 in the household
75 percent are adults without children under 18 in the household
81 percent are adults employed full-time
77 percent are adults employed part-time
68 percent are adults without employment
76 percent are retired adults
81 percent are adults who are married
73 percent are adults who live in the Northeast
74 percent are adults who live in the Midwest
80 percent are adults who live in the South
78 percent are adults who live in the West

Although most experts say we do not need supplements to be healthy, CRN's 2020 survey found that vitamins & minerals continue to be the most commonly consumed supplement, with 76 percent of Americans consuming them. Specialty supplements at 40 percent were in second place, third by herbals and botanicals at 39 percent, fourth by sports nutrition supplements at 28 percent, and weight management supplements at 17 percent (www.crnusa.org). People can feel that their bodies are out of balance and are actively seeking to rebalance themselves with supplementation.

4. Who is deficient and who needs supplements?

I recommended to my patient to exercise to slim down as well as some orange juice for vitamins. He said, "It's the weight and C approach I guess?"

Most of us see someone overweight and assume they are most likely getting too much nutrition and that's why they're overweight. In fact the opposite is actually true, an obese person can be just as malnourished as an extremely thin person. Being deficient in vitamins can lead to adverse weight effects.

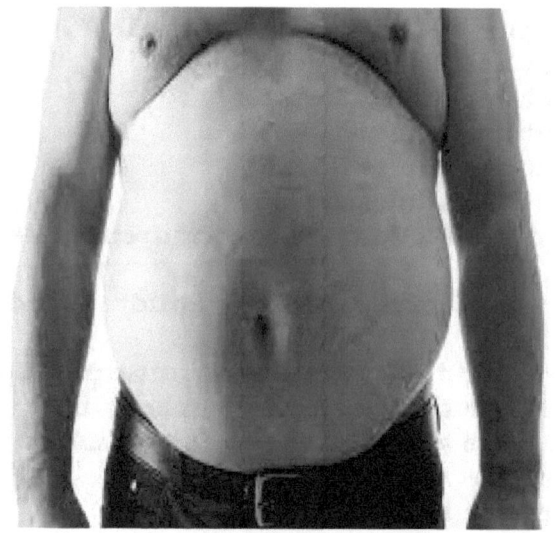

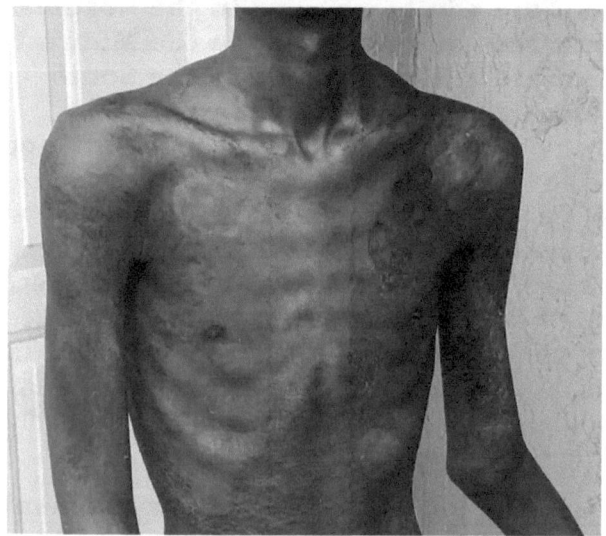

Nutrient deficiencies exist in 92 percent of the U.S. population regardless of socioeconomic background. According to the recommended dietary intake, the country is overfed and undernourished. Even if you consume a "perfect" diet, you are probably deficient in at least one vitamin or mineral.

Some of the groups most prone to nutrient deficiencies are

A. Pregnant Women.

Prenatal vitamins with folic acid are recommended for all pregnant women or planning on becoming pregnant. Iron is another nutrient often deficient in pregnant women, especially if you get morning sickness.

B. Infants and Children.

Infants and children often need supplementation for vitamin D and iron.

C. Those on Restrictive Diets

People who eat a restricted or limited diet, such as vegans or people with a dairy allergy, often struggle to get enough vitamin B12 or calcium.

D. Adults Over 50

Adults over 50 start to absorb fewer vitamins D and B12, so they may need extra supplementation to get enough.

E. Bypass Surgery Recipients

If you've had gastric bypass surgery. Your gut may not absorb nutrients as well, so you'll need supplementation.

F. Those with Malabsorption of Nutrients

Some people have genetic or health conditions that affect the absorption of nutrients.

G. Those with Inflammatory Diseases such as:

Ulcerative Colitis
Crohn's Disease
Celiac disease
Cystic fibrosis
Liver disease
Cancer
An autoimmune disorder (ie. pernicious anemia)

H. Other Factors such as:

Darker skin (decreased ability to absorb Vitamin D)
Alcohol dependence
A mutation in specific genes

5. Do supplements work?

During a trip to Medellin, Colombia, I met Ana, who shared that she had been experiencing migraines. Her headaches were so debilitating that she often had to miss several workdays when they randomly appeared. After years of trying multiple prescription medications with no success, she accepted headaches as part of her life. She was forced to live at the will of her migraines, limiting her activities and, if they were terrible enough, staying home and missing several days of work, putting her in financial binds. After hearing about Ana's migraines, I referenced a National Institute of Health (NIH) study that said 40% of migraine study participants who took magnesium saw an improvement in their symptoms. After gifting her a bottle of magnesium citrate, her migraines disappeared, and after several years she has not had another migraine.

Magnesium is an example of a nutrient vital to your health. Yet, it is challenging to consume a consistent quantity through diet alone. It's found in foods such as pumpkin seeds, almonds, spinach, and cashews. Foods that most people don't have access to regularly.

Most researchers agree that popping dietary supplements will not solve most people's health problems, and you'd be better off investing your money in nutritious foods.

Researchers found that vitamins A, K, magnesium, zinc, and copper consumption were linked to a lower risk of death from heart disease, stroke, and an overall lower risk of dying when the nutrients came from foods, not supplements.

They also found that overdosing on some supplements, such as 1,000 milligrams of calcium daily, increased your risk of death, but the same is not true of calcium from food.

Supplements can not make up for not eating a healthy balanced diet. One of the reasons why supplements can not give you the same benefits as eating whole foods is that nutrients typically come in groups. For example, broccoli contains calcium, iron, phosphorous, potassium, zinc, thiamin, riboflavin, niacin, vitamins A, B6, B12, D, E, and K, folate, lipophilic phytonutrients, including; carotenoids lutein, zeaxanthin, β-carotene, and tocopherols, (forms of vitamin E). Many of these nutrients work synergistically for absorption and health benefits, and when they are separated, the benefits are just not as profound. It is also much easier for the body to regulate and limit the absorption of nutrients from whole foods versus supplements. Eat your veggies!

However, most of the studies conducted are on healthy people who tend to eat healthier diets. Study participants were also tested for certain nutrients, not all. For example, almost everyone is deficient in vitamin D, and people living a vegan lifestyle may come up short on vitamin B12, vitamin D, and omega-3 fatty acids. Therefore people who don't eat healthy diets would most likely benefit from supplements. Supplements will not solve your health issues. But there are times when supplementation with vitamins or minerals can help you.

Although supplements can be helpful, people feel that if a little is good, more is better. Our bodies work to maintain a very delicate balance, and taking too much of a nutrient can knock that balance off causing a deficiency in other nutrients.

No supplement can include all the vital plant compounds in fruits and vegetables, legumes, nuts and seeds, and whole grains. The nutrients in foods work synergistically to help keep us fighting disease and staying healthy.

Based on anecdotal evidence, I've witnessed patients whose health is dramatically improved by simply giving their bodies supplements they lacked. Benefits such as increased energy, improved cognitive function, and weight loss, for example. After reading a study by the National Institute of Health (NIH) about the effectiveness of taking magnesium for treating migraines, I started recommending it to my patients. Although the study stated that over 40% of study participants saw improvements in their migraines, I've seen a 75% improvement in my patients. In my opinion, nutritional supplementation is undervalued and underutilized in our healthcare system. In 440 BC, the famous Greek physician Hippocrates said, "Let food be thy medicine and let thy medicine be food," 2,383 years after his death, people are starting to believe he was right.

Scientific evidence, however, isn't unequivocal despite the amount of research done on supplements, The National Institutes of Health (NIH) has spent more than $2.4 billion studying minerals and vitamins since 1999. Most studies suggest that multivitamins won't improve your health very much (However a properly dosed multivitamin formulated for your sex and age group have been shown to be more effective). It's also illegal for companies to make such claims about supplements' ability to treat, diagnose, prevent or cure diseases. Keep in mind that the products you buy in stores or online may be different from those used in studies, so the results from the studies may not match actual outcomes.

6. Some supplements that can cause health risks include:

I just took a part-time job at a vitamin store... for some supplemental income.

In most cases, supplements aren't likely to pose any health risks, yet it's best to be cautious when you put anything into your body. Supplements may interact with other medications for specific medical conditions, such as liver disease, or interfere with surgery; and children, pregnant women, and nursing mothers should take extra precautions. Federal regulations for dietary supplements are less strict than prescription drugs. Some products sold as nutritional supplements can have prescription drugs included which are not listed in the ingredients, which can be unsafe.

Beta-carotene and vitamin A can increase the risk of lung cancer in smokers.

Vitamin K can reduce the effectiveness of blood thinners.

Vitamins D and K should be taken together because they help the body use calcium optimally for building bone instead of depositing it dangerously in arteries and soft tissue.

St. John's wort can decrease the effectiveness of antidepressants and birth control.

Gingko Biloba can increase blood thinning.

Comfrey and kava can damage your liver.

Speak with your healthcare provider before taking any supplements. Since our bodies are unique and have individual needs, it's best to discuss your options with your healthcare provider since a supplement's effectiveness and safety can depend on your needs.

Some simple safety tips to keep in mind as you choose a supplement:

A. Take supplements as directed by the label and your healthcare provider's instructions.

B. Be aware of the ingredients, drug interactions, and percent daily value (% DV) of your supplement.

C. Be cautious of health claims and remember that "natural" doesn't mean safe.

D. Keep supplements appropriately stored and away from children.

E. Read about the potential dangers of the supplement.

Supplements cannot replace a healthy diet. So never take supplements in place of eating a healthy meal. Supplements are meant to be supplementary. Which means they enhance the benefits of eating a healthy diet. Vitamins and minerals are essential to good health. Supplements can help support your body's needs to stay healthy.

7. Dietary Supplement Labels

What kind of vitamin improves your eyesight? Vitamin see!

DSHEA and federal regulations require the following information to be printed on dietary supplement labels: a statement of identity containing "dietary supplement." The supplement label has printed, written, or graphic material on the supplement container. The term "dietary" may be replaced by the name of the dietary ingredient (e.g., "green tea supplement"), quantity of contents (i.e., "50 capsules"), nutrition information on the "Supplement Facts" panel, including the amount, product serving size, and percent daily value, if established, of each dietary ingredient. If the supplement contains a proprietary blend, it must have the net weight of the combination and a listing of each component from highest concentration to lowest in descending order, weight, if an herb or botanical (part of the plant used must be identified), name and place of business of the manufacturer, packer, or distributor, and a complete list of ingredients by their common or usual names.

The "Supplement Facts" panel follows the name of the dietary ingredient, safety information that is considered "material" to the consequences that may result from the use of the supplement, the disclaimer "The Food and Drug Administration has not evaluated this statement. This product is not intended to diagnose, treat, cure, or prevent any disease," must appear if the product is claiming a health benefit. The manufacturers may also provide additional information on labels (such as claims and statements of quality assurance) and decide on the placement of that information on their labels.

8. Relationship between Nutrition and Disease.

A bumblebee, a spelling bee and a vitamin B got in a fight. "The vitamin B1."

Researchers show that eating too much or not enough nutrient-dense foods can raise the risk of dying of a stroke, heart disease, and type 2 diabetes. Changing eating habits may help improve health and prevent disease.

Eating healthy can lower your risk of stroke, heart disease, diabetes, and other cardiometabolic diseases. A healthy diet consists of whole grains, fat-free or low-fat dairy products, fruits, vegetables, beans, eggs, nuts, limited lean meats, poultry, fish, saturated and trans fats, sodium, and added sugars. Consuming too much salt, sugar, or fat can increase your risk for disease.

Almost half of all deaths in the United States caused by cardiometabolic diseases (heart disease, type 2 diabetes, and stroke) are due to poor eating habits. The highest percentage of cardiometabolic disease-related death is caused by excess salt consumption (9.5%). Not eating enough seeds and nuts (8.5%), seafood or plant-based omega-3 fats (7.8%), vegetables (7.6%), fruits (7.5%), whole grains (5.9%), or polyunsaturated fats (2.3%) also increased the risk of death compared with people who had an optimal intake of these foods/nutrients. Overeating processed meat (8.2%), sugary beverages (7.4%), and unprocessed red meat (0.4%) also raised the risk of stroke, heart disease, stroke, and type 2 diabetes-related deaths. The highest death levels were amongst men, blacks, Hispanics, and people with lower education levels.

9. Nutritional Approach to Health

I discovered the cure for blindness. "Vitamin See"

As our food environment continues to decline, people become more susceptible to environmental damage from food.

As Hippocrates said in 400 BC, "Let thy food be thy medicine and medicine be thy food," and emphasized the importance of nutrition to prevent or cure disease.

Nutritional therapy is the promotion of health through personalized nutrition and lifestyle support. A whole-body approach to lifestyle medicine and nutrition addresses the potential underlying causes of ill-health rather than focusing on symptoms.

Four factors to consider when developing your nutritional approach are:

1 Enjoyment – taking satisfaction in the sensory pleasure of food (aroma, appearance, texture, taste)

2 Connection – the role of nutrition in relationships, culture, faith, ritual, tradition, self-expression

3 Social justice – food security (access to affordable, safe, culturally appropriate food), sustainability

4 Food as medicine – therapeutic diet strategies to address medical conditions

10. As the World Ages the Need for Supplements Increases.

Worldwide, people over 65 years old increased from 6 percent in 1990 to 9 percent in 2019. This group is expected to increase to 16 percent by 2050, so one in six people in the world will be over 65 years old. The older people get, the more susceptible they are to nutritional deficiencies, causing an embrace in dietary supplements as people search for alternatives to increase their quality of life and decrease their dependence on allopathic medicine. (www.un.org)

11. What are Vitamins?

What is the tumor's favorite vitamin? It's B-9.

To both survive and thrive, the human body depends on vitamins. All of them have a specific purpose, and they're all crucial. The body requires 13 essential vitamins to thrive, including:

Vitamin A

Vitamin B1 (thiamine)
Vitamin B2 (riboflavin)
Vitamin B3 (niacin)
Vitamin B5 (pantothenic acid)
Vitamin B6 (pyridoxine)
Vitamin B7 (biotin)
Vitamin B9 (folate or folic acid)
Vitamin B12 (cyanocobalamin)
Vitamin C
Vitamin D
Vitamin E
Vitamin K

Nutrient	Function	Signs and Symptoms of Deficiency
Vitamin A	Involved in immune function, vision, cell growth and cell communication.	Night blindness and xerophthalmia
Vitamin B6	Involved in greater than 100 enzyme reactions in the body and involved in protein metabolism.	Microcytic anemia, scaling of the lips and cracks in the corners of the mouth, swollen tongue, depression, and confusion
Vitamin B12	Involved in red blood cell formation, neurological function, and DNA synthesis	Megaloblastic anemia, fatigue, weakness, constipation, loss of appetite, and weight loss
Vitamin C	Involved in the formation of collagen, certain neurotransmitters, and protein synthesis.	Development of scurvy which would include: fatigue, inflammation of the gums, and weakened connective tissue
Vitamin D	Promotes calcium	Development of

Nutrient	Function	Signs and Symptoms of Deficiency
	absorption and proper bone formation, involved in cell growth, immune function, and reduces inflammation	rickets in children or osteomalacia in adults, and fatigue
Calcium	Involved in muscle function, nerve transmission, and proper bone formation.	Development of osteoporosis
Folate	Involved in the synthesis of RNA and DNA and is required for cell division and the prevention of Neural Tube Defects.	Megaloblastic anemia
Iodine	A component of thyroid hormones that regulate protein synthesis, metabolism, and enzyme activity.	Stunted growth and neurodevelopmental deficits
Iron	A component of hemoglobin and therefore important in the transfer of oxygen from the lungs to organs, and involved in the synthesis of hormones as well as normal growth and development.	Microcytic, hypochromic anemia; impaired cognitive function, poor body temperature regulation, depressed immune function, and spoon like shape of nails
Magnesium	Involved in more than 300 enzyme	Loss of appetite, fatigue, weakness,

Nutrient	Function	Signs and Symptoms of Deficiency
	reactions, protein synthesis, muscle function, nerve function, blood sugar control, and blood pressure control.	nausea, vomiting, numbness, tingling, muscle cramps, seizures, personality changes, and abnormal heart rhythms
Zinc	Involved in cell metabolism, enzyme activity, immune function, protein synthesis, wound healing, DNA synthesis, and cell division	Stunted growth, depressed immune function, hair loss, eye and skin lesions, delayed wound healing, and taste alterations

12. Can I get my vitamins from my diet?

Theoretically, you can get these essential vitamins from the foods you eat. Not eating enough vitamin-rich foods can lead to several health-related issues, including unhealthy bones, disease, mouth ulcers, and hair loss. Vitamin deficiency can also cause other symptoms like dizziness, cognitive decline, neurological problems, and many more. A lack of vitamins causes these health problems. They mainly serve as catalysts for specific reactions in the body. These are some of the foods you should be eating daily to maintain healthy vitamin levels:

Fruits
Nuts
Legumes
Vegetables
Whole grains

Because fewer people eat these foods in their unprocessed form daily, along with many other factors (lack of sunlight, pollution, soil nutrient depletion, chronic diseases, or nutritional absorption issues), supplements may be an excellent way to fill in any gaps in your nutrition.

Dr. Mark Fuhrman developed The Aggregate Nutrient Density Index Scores (ANDI) to help people select a nutrient-dense diet and lose weight faster. Dr. Fuhrman created this simple formula:

H= N/C (Health = Nutrients divided by Calories.

The equation demonstrates how health is affected by the nutrient density of your diet. Sufficient consumption of micronutrients – vitamins, minerals, and many other phytochemicals – is the key to achieving excellent health without excessive caloric intake.

The ANDI is a ranking of common foods and how many nutrients you should expect to be delivered to your body by eating them. It's a quick reference guide to which foods have the highest nutrient-per-calorie density, the most health-promoting, and nutrient-dense. The ANDI uses 34 nutritional parameters, unlike food labels that list only a few nutrients. Foods on the scale are ranked from 1-to 1000, with the most nutrient-dense vegetables scoring 1000.

Eating various plant foods is crucial to obtaining a full range of nutritional requirements. It is also vital to achieving micronutrient diversity, not just a high level of a few isolated micronutrients. They all contribute to the numerator (the top number in the ratio) in the H=N/C equation.

VEGETABLES	
Kale & Collard Greens (1.5 cups)	1000
Bok Choy (1.5 cups)	824
Spinach, Raw (5 cups)	739
Chinese/Napa Cabbage, (1.5 cups)	704
Spinach, cooked (1.5 cups)	697
Brussel Sprouts, cooked (1.5 cups)	672
Arugula, raw (5 cups)	559
Radish (6 items)	554
Bean Sprouts, uncooked (1 cup)	444
Cabbage, raw (1.5 cups)	420
Lettuce, Romaine (5 cups)	389
Broccoli, raw (1.5 cups)	376
Pepper, red, cooked (1.5 cups)	366
Turnips, cooked (1 item)	337
Carrots, cooked (1.5 cups)	336
Pepper, red, raw (1.5 cups)	328
Mixed Baby Greens (5 cups)	300
Cauliflower, cooked (1.5 cups)	295
Pepper, green, raw (1.5 cups)	258
Artichoke, cooked (1 item)	244
Asparagus, cooked (1.5 cups)	234
Zucchini, raw (2.5 cups)	209
Tomato, raw (1 item)	164
Butternut Squash, (1.5 cups)	156
Eggplant, cooked (1.5 cups)	149
Bamboo shoots, canned (1 cup)	144
Okra, cooked (1.5 cups)	139
Celery (2 items)	135
Alfalfa Sprouts (1 cup)	130
Snow or sugar peas, raw (1.5 cups)	127

Mushrooms, cooked (1.5 cups)	119
Lettuce, Iceberg (5 cups)	110
Beets, cooked (1.5 cups)	97
Sweet Potato, cooked (1.5 cups)	83
Green Beans, cooked (2 cups)	74
Green Peas, cooked (1.5 cups)	70
Cucumber (1 item)	50
Onions, cooked (.33 cups)	50
Spaghetti & Acorn Squash, (1.5 cups)	49
Corn, sweet, white, (1.5 cups)	44
Potatoes, baked w/skin (1 item)	43
Yams, cooked (1.5 cups)	23
Olives (3 items)	24
FRUITS	
Strawberries (1.5 cups)	212
Blackberries (1.5 cups)	178
Plums (1.5 cups)	157
Raspberries (1.5 cups)	145
Blueberries (1.5 cups)	130
Papaya (1.5 cups)	118
Orange & Grapefruit (1.5 cups)	105
Cantaloupe (1.5 cups)	100
Kiwi (2 items)	97
Watermelon (2.5 cups)	91
Peach, Apple & Tangerine (1 item)	73
Cherries (1.5 cups)	68
Pineapple (1.5 cups)	64
Apricots fresh (4 items)	60
Mango (1 item)	51
Prunes (.25 cup)	47
Pears (1 item)	46

Honeydew (1.5 cups)	45
Nectarine (1.5 cups)	41
Avocado (half)	37
Cranberries, dried, (.33 cup)	34
Grapes (1.5 cups)	31
Banana (1 item)	30
Apricots, dried, (.33 cup)	29
Figs, dried (.25 cup)	25
Dates & Raisins (.25 cup)	18
JUICES	
Vegetable Juice, regular (8 fl oz)	365
Carrot Juice (8 fl oz)	344
Tomato Juice, regular (8 fl oz)	342
Pomegranate Juice (8 fl oz)	193
Orange Juice (8 fl oz)	86
Cranberry Juice Cocktail (8 fl oz)	55
Apple Juice, unsweetened (8 fl oz)	16
BEANS	
Lentils, boiled (1 cup)	104
Red Kidney Beans, boiled (1 cup)	100
Great Northern Beans, (1 cup)	94
Adzuki Beans, boiled (1 cup)	84
Black beans & Black Eyed Peas, (1 cup)	83
Hummus (.5 cup)	70
Pinto Beans, boiled (1 cup)	61
Edamame (1 cup)	58
Split Peas, boiled (1 cup)	58
Chick Peas/Garbanzo bean, (1 cup)	57
Lima Beans, boiled (1 cup)	46
Tofu (4 oz)	37
Tempeh (4 oz)	26

NUTS	
Brazil Nuts & Pecans (.25 cup)	124
Pistachio Nuts, unsalted (.25 cup)	48
Almonds & Peanuts, unsalted (.25 cup)	38
Walnuts (.25 cup)	34
Hazelnuts or filberts (.25 cup)	32
Cashew Nuts, unsalted (.25 cup)	27
Pine Nuts/Pignolia (1 tbsp)	26
Macadamia nuts, unsalted (.25 cup)	17
NUT BUTTERS	
Tahini & Sesame Butter (2 tbsp)	54
Almond, Cashew & Peanut Butter (2 tbsp)	26
SEEDS	
Sunflower Seeds (.25 cup)	78
Flax Seeds & Sesame Seeds (2 tbsp)	65
Pumpkin Seeds (.25 cup)	52
GRAINS	
Bran Flakes (1 cup)	64
Oats, old fashioned, (1 cup)	53
Barley, whole grain, (1 cup)	43
Wild Rice, cooked (1 cup)	43
Brown Rice, cooked (1 cup)	41
Sprouted Grain Bread (1 slice)	39
Whole Grain Bread (2 slices)	30
Whole Wheat Bagel (1 item)	25
Granola (1 cup)	22
Cornmeal, whole grain (.25 cup)	22
Quinoa, cooked (1 cup)	21
Rye Bread (2 slices)	20
Whole Wheat Pasta, cooked (1 cup)	19
Oats, quick, cooked (1 cup)	19

White Bread (2 slices) & White Pasta, (1 cup)	18	Cheese, hard (2 oz)	15
Couscous, cooked (1 cup)	15	Cottage Cheese (1 cup)	13
Tortilla, flour/corn (2 items, 52g)	14	Ice Cream/ Frozen Yogurt (1 cup)	9
White Rice (1 c) & Rice Cakes (7 pieces)	12	**DAIRY SUBSTITUTES**	
Saltines (5 items)	11	Soy Milk (8 fl oz)	33
Graham Crackers (2 1/2" squares)	8	Almond Milk (8 fl oz)	19
SEAFOOD		Rice Milk (8 fl oz)	10
Shrimp, cooked (4 oz)	48	**FAST FOOD**	
Tuna, yellow fin, cooked, (4 oz)	46	Cheese Pizza (2 slices)	17
Lobster, cooked (4 oz)	43	Biscuit w/ Egg & Bacon, (1 item)	11
Flounder, cooked, dry heat (4 oz)	41	Fast Food Cheeseburger (1 item)	11
Salmon & Mahi-Mahi, cooked, (4 oz)	39	Fish Filet, Batter Coated, Fried (4 oz)	7
Swordfish, cooked, dry heat (4 oz)	38	French Fried Potatoes, (2.5 oz)	7
Tuna, in water (4 oz)	36	**SNACK FOODS**	
Snapper, cooked, dry heat (4 oz)	35	Dark Chocolate Candy Bar (1.5 oz)	34
Cod & Grouper, cooked, dry heat (4 oz)	31	Milk Chocolate Candy Bar (1.5 oz)	21
Scallops, steamed (4 oz)	24	Popcorn, air popped, no salt (4 cups)	16
Tilapia, cooked, dry heat (4 oz)	18	Hard pretzels, salted (10 items, 60g)	13
MEAT		Fruit Roll Ups (1 item)	12
Bison, top sirloin, broiled (4 oz)	39	Chocolate Pudding (1 cup)	11
Chicken Breast, roasted (4 oz)	27	Granola Bar (1 item)	11
Egg (1 item)	27	Potato Chips & Corn Chips, (1 oz)	10
Pork Loin, Whole, roasted (4 oz)	23	Toaster Pastry (1 item) & Fig Bar (2 items)	8
Beef Top Sirloin, 1/8" fat (4 oz)	20	Popcorn, oil popped, no salt (4 cups)	8
Ham, Boneless, roasted & Lamb (4 oz)	17	Corn Puffs, cheese flavored (1 oz)	8
Bacon & Bologna (2 oz) & Sausage (4 oz)	14	Chocolate chip cookies, ready to eat (3)	7
DAIRY		Apple Pie, Prepared (1 slice)	6
Milk, low fat 1% (8 oz)	28	Chocolate Cake with frosting (1 slice)	5
Plain Yogurt, low fat (1 cup)	24	**ALCOHOL**	
Chocolate Milk (8 oz)	19	Beer (12 fluid ounces)	7
Fruit Yogurt, low fat (1 cup)	15	Wine (4 fluid ounces)	3

13. How are Vitamins and Supplements Made?

Why did Vladimir Putin (the Russian leader of an oppressive regime) start taking vitamin pills in abundance? Because there were too many free radicals.

Supplements are made from plant or animal products. For example, vitamin A can be synthesized from leafy green vegetables, orange and yellow vegetables, tomato products, fruits, or vegetable oils. Regardless of what it is extracted from, there should be no structural difference in the supplement.

There are many steps in making a vitamin. A vitamin manufacturer will buy raw vitamins and other ingredients from distributors. Then they will process it and blend it as requested by the retailer. Some steps may include a wet granulation stage, which helps the vitamin be sized appropriately. They are weighed and then correctly dispensed. For example, a specific amount of powder is put into each capsule at this stage. Then polished, cleaned of dust or debris, and inspected. The vitamin manufacturing process will change, depending on the form of the vitamin, i.e., tablet, pill, or coated. There are quality control checks at several steps in the process at several different stages.

14. How to Differentiate Between Herbal Products?

Herbal medicines are becoming mainstream, and many forms of the same herbal supplement are available. The most important decision is whether to use standardized herbal extracts or whole herbs. The easiest way to decide is to know the difference between the two to make an informed decision.

While backpacking in South America, we visited native tribes in every country. We watched as the Shaman gathered plants from the forest to brew a fresh batch of Ayahuasca, a plant-based psychedelic that indigenous people have used as a healing medicine, and as part of religious ceremonies and tribal rituals for thousands of years. Psychedelics affect all the senses, altering a person's thinking, understanding of time, and emotions. They can cause a person to hallucinate seeing or hearing things that do not exist. They use it to treat physical and mental problems and deal with spiritual crises.

I brought my cousin, an Iraq war veteran, with me to try an ayahuasca treatment on one trip. He described the experience as healing and feeling like he had football pads removed from his body. I saw him again several months later, and he had lost weight; his face glowed, and he was enrolled in college, taking five courses.

Standardized Herbal Extract

What do you say when you don't have enough vitamin D? Vitamin d-ficient.

Standardization of herbs guarantees that the consumer gets a chemically consistent product from batch to batch. A standardized herbal extract has one or more components in a specific, confirmed amount, usually expressed as a percentage. Modern scientists have developed the drug model of herbal medicine to identify the components of a plant that have pharmacological activity in the body. Scientists can isolate many chemicals from an herb and discover how they act in the body. However, they sometimes accidentally overlook or remove components that affect the function of the whole herb. Therefore, standardization may concentrate one constituent at the expense of other potentially important ones while changing the natural balance of the herb's components.

The medicinal value of an herb is determined by its composition and the interactions of the different components within the body rather than one of its specific components. Standardization is based on the idea that isolated compounds are responsible for the action of an herb. However, almost no medicinal herbs are known for just a single function. Plants are made up of a complex blend of phytochemicals, and naturally concentrated foods have the unique ability to address a diversity of problems simultaneously. Many of an herb's constituents are unknown, and internal chemical interactions within and among herbs are less understood. Therefore, standardized herbal extract can not exhibit the same full spectrum of benefits as the whole herb. However, science has proven that some of these concentrated extracts can be beneficial even if they don't work exactly like the entire herb.

The second form of standardization only uses key components as identity markers while maintaining the same full spectrum of components as the herb. These standardized extracts are not more concentrated than the whole herbs, but they hold a minimum potency of these markers. The markers can or can not be active plant constituents. Still, spectrum analysis of this kind of extract should be visually similar to the whole herb, assuring that no vital components have been removed in the extraction process. They promise that the herbs will have a minimum potency level every time without sacrificing any components.

My grandfather Dr. Baudelio Medina was a gynecologist in Los Angeles, delivering thousands of babies over his forty years of practicing medicine. His office was full of jars of different herbs, and as part of his practice, he relied heavily on herbs to treat various health problems. He believed, as I do, that instead of always using pharmaceuticals derived from herbs, you could use the herbs themselves with better outcomes and fewer side effects.

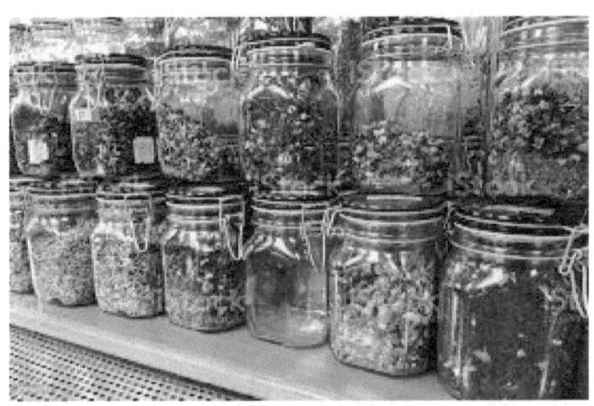

Whole Herbs
What's a Canadian's favorite vitamin? Eh

A whole herb is usually dried, encapsulated, processed, and preserved in alcohol or another solvent. Whole herbs contain all of the plant's constituents and represent the most common use of most plants for hundreds of years by many cultures. Whole herbs have been used to make most modern medicines. The medicinal properties of herbs have been discovered through empirical observation, and the information has been passed down through generations of healers. Although the effects of herbs have not always been formally and scientifically researched, whole herbs have a long track record validating their safety and efficacy.

An herb's chemical makeup can vary depending on a variety of factors:
1. The plant's growing environment affects the herb's constituents. Also, the time of year it is harvested, the soil in which it is grown, and the weather influence the final product's overall quality.
2. The age of the herb at harvest, the part of the plant being used, and processing techniques can all make a difference.
3. Each plant or population has its genetics, thus adding another source of end-product variation.

My father is originally from Mexico, and he always had a pot of beans on the stove. One of his secret ingredients was the herb epazote. When cooked with beans, this herb reduces flatulence. You will have gas if you don't soak your beans overnight or use the herb epazote when cooking beans.

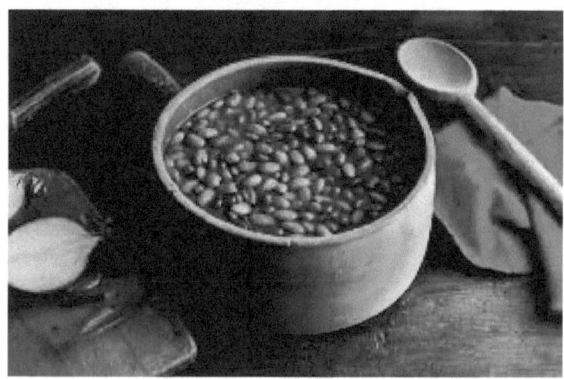

Active versus Marker Compounds

An active compound is a plant constituent that exerts a direct physiological effect. A marker compound is a constituent useful for technical purposes, but that does not necessarily exert a physiological influence.

Marker compounds are selected for special attention by a researcher or manufacturer. The marker compound is chosen based on the availability of analytical methods and standards, ease of analysis, value in identifying the botanical material, use as an indicator of quality and stability, health relevance, and previous use of a marker compound by different manufacturers. The compound levels are quantitatively determined in both raw materials and products and are used as a guide for manufacturing the product.

15. What is the Difference Between Concentrated and Standardized Extracts?

Powdered herb extracts come in two forms: concentrated and standardized powdered extract. Because these two products are similar and look similar, most people do not consider the differences. However, it is vital to understand how the differences affect the final product.

First, know that powdered extracts are potent, shelf-stable extracts of medicinal herbs, fungi, and animal products. They dissolve quickly in water and are easy to use. Most even have a pleasant flavor. It is common to have powdered extracts that are ten times the concentration of the plant, whereas most liquid extracts (i.e., tinctures) are a four or five times dilution of the plant (which is the opposite of an extract).

Concentrated Powdered Extracts

The concentrated powdered extract is made of the original herb and water (sometimes alcohol is used). The mixture is cooked until the aspired concentration is reached, and then it is spray dried. Then it is marked with the concentration ratio, which is usually a 5:1 or a 10:1. A 10:1 extract concentration means that ten parts of the original plant produced one part of the final extract, resulting in a concentrated product. Remember, taking one teaspoon of powdered extract equals three tablespoons of the whole herb.

Standardized Powdered Extracts

The active polysaccharides are concentrated with extracts of medicinal fungi, as in our Chaga, Reishi, and Turkey Tail extracts. Standardized powdered extracts are made similar to concentrated extracts, except that the mixture of herb and water (or alcohol) is heated and reduced to an exact concentration of the desired compound. Resulting in a highly concentrated extract, as high as 30:1 extract (or beyond) is reached with a standardized extract.

Standardized extracts are more concentrated than most other powdered extracts and provide unique information of the actual content of identified, active medicinal compounds in plants. These compounds can vary widely, depending on many factors, including growing region, soil conditions, and harvest time. Knowing exactly how much of a particular compound is in the extract you are taking is valuable, especially for prescribing herbalists.

16. How are Dietary Supplements Tested?

I would like vitamins for my son, a mother said.
Vitamin A, B or C? the pharmacist asked.

It doesn't matter, the mother replied. He can't read yet.

Three Stages of Dietary Supplement Testing

Dietary supplement manufacturers must follow a strict and consistent quality control process to deliver safe and quality products to consumers. Manufacturers test every product for quality, safety, efficacy, and stability by testing identity, purity, strength, and composition throughout the process. They help assure the manufacturer that the finished product will be safe for human consumption and that every batch is accurate to its supplement facts and marketed quality. The dietary supplement product testing process should include three lab and testing stages: raw material testing, finished product testing, and stability testing.

A. Raw Material Testing

Manufacturers will conduct raw material testing in the first stage of the dietary supplement product testing process. Each raw material is tested for identity, purity, and strength specifications. Materials must also be tested for their composition related to incoming components and types of contaminants that may degrade the finished product. Manufacturers must also perform identity testing of all incoming ingredients, using fully validated chromatographic and spectroscopic methods. After completing this testing stage and verifying that each specification has been met, the raw materials will be approved for integration into the dietary supplement.

B. Finished Product Testing

Finished product testing is the second stage in the dietary supplement testing process. Manufacturers will conduct finished product testing after raw material testing and manufacturing of each dietary supplement batch. Each batch of the finished product is tested to verify that it meets each product specification for identity, purity, strength, composition, and limits on contamination. Consumers should have confidence in what they are taking and that the supplement facts are not misleading in any way. Every dietary ingredient listed on the Supplement Facts Panel (SFP) is addressed on the finished product specification. Each must have an appropriate minimum test acceptance criterion that meets each product specification for identity, purity, strength, composition, and limits on contamination. After each finished batch is thoroughly tested for quality and safety, they are tested again for stability.

C. Stability Testing

Manufacturers will complete stability testing in the third stage of the dietary supplement product testing process. The purpose of stability testing is to verify that no unexpected organoleptic changes occur during the period of the proposed shelf life for the product. Also, to ensure that the dietary supplement still meets the supplement facts and requirements for the claimed active ingredients throughout that time. This verified testing allows the manufacturer to predict a suitable shelf life to meet consumer expectations. The stability of dietary supplements may be affected by environmental factors (i.e., oxygen, temperature, moisture), pH level, water activity, oxidization, and metallic ions. Once the last stage of the dietary supplement product testing is completed, a Certificate of Analysis for that dietary supplement is created to ensure the retailer or wholesaler of its verification.

Every dietary supplement manufactured should undergo these three important lab and testing stages: raw material testing, finished product testing, and stability testing. Some manufacturers may outsource some dietary supplement product testing while others run all their raw material, finished product, and stability testing in-house. The manufacturer's dietary supplement product testing process is meant to increase the safety of dietary supplements, match consumer expectations, and meet product requirements. Using trained chemists and biologists, this is performed using fully validated methods on qualified and certified equipment, including heavy metal, microbiological, and strength/composition tests. A Certificate of Analysis should always back this.

17. How to Spot Fraudulent Products?

Nutritional supplements don't usually have health warnings on them, but that's what you should be thinking about when you see grandiose health claims. Health scams have been around for a very long time and play on people's desire for a quick or miracle cure. The snake-oil salesmen of the past have transformed into high-tech marketers. They prey on people's desires for easy solutions to health problems such as coronavirus, Alzheimer's, arthritis, diabetes, memory loss, cancer, sexual performance, weight loss, and other infectious diseases. The Food and Drug Administration (FDA) views any health product as fraudulent if it is deceptively promoted as effective against a health condition or disease, without any scientific evidence to support its claim.

Social media is the most popular place for health fraud scammers to spread misinformation and rob people. Scammers promote their products with deceptive marketing that targets specific populations via the web, email, word-of-mouth, newspapers, TV, magazines, and direct mail. However, scammers also operate in convenience stores, gas stations, flea markets, and nontraditional stores, targeting people with limited English proficiency, limited access to health care services, and information. Some products are also marketed overseas via mail to circumvent typical FDA and Customs inspections and other safety measures.

18. How to avoid supplement Scams?

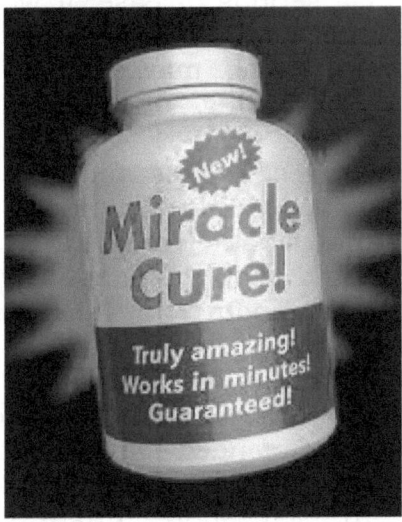

1. One product does it all. Be careful of products that claim to cure a wide range of diseases. Miracle cures don't exist, they're bogus, and the only thing these companies are selling is false hope.
2. Personal "success" testimonials. Reviews found on online marketplaces and social media are often fake. Success stories are easy to make up and are not substitutes for scientific evidence.
3. Quick fixes. Even with legitimate products, few diseases or conditions can be treated quickly. Beware of language such as "fast weight loss that works" or "prevent or treat heart disease, prostate cancer, and erectile dysfunction."
4. "All-natural" cure or treatment. Be skeptical of such phrases often used as attention-grabbers to suggest safer products than conventional treatments. Natural doesn't equate to safety. Some plants found in nature (such as poisonous mushrooms) can kill or be harmful when consumed. Some products labeled as all-natural contain hidden and dangerously high doses of prescription drug ingredients or other active pharmaceutical ingredients.
5. "Miracle cure." Question, when you see claims, such as "guaranteed results," "new discovery," or "secret

ingredient." If a groundbreaking discovery had been made to treat a serious disease, it would be prescribed by licensed health professionals and reported through the media, not being marketed on websites, social media, and messaging apps, print ads, and TV infomercials.
6. Conspiracy theories. Claims such as "This is the cure our government or pharmaceutical companies don't want you to know about" are used to attract people that are skeptical and distract consumers from common-sense questions about the so-called miracle cure (www.fda.gov).
7. Underdosing. Marketing a supplement and then purposely creating a product that provides much less than the recommended daily allowance of the supplement to increase profit margins and decrease the sale price to sell more quantity. When buying supplements, make sure that you check the recommended daily allowances for each desired ingredient and compare that number to the product you're considering purchasing.
8. Adulteration. The process of substituting expensive ingredients for cheap ones to increase profit margins. For example, the herb Goldenseal is much more costly when buying the leaf with a higher active ingredient potency. But to save money, some manufacturers will use more stems in the supplement with a lower potency. Some manufacturers may also substitute an entirely different, less expensive supplement but still market the original product.
9. Bait and switch. Sometimes the manufacturer sends a high-quality sample to the lab for quality testing. But when they actually produce the product, they use something much lower in quality and less expensive to increase profit margin.

Be careful as unregistered facilities manufacture fraudulent products under unknown, unclean, or dangerous conditions. Many of these products are mixed with pharmaceutical drugs that can cause heart attack and stroke.

Even still, it's hard to spot fraudulent health products. If you're tempted to buy an unproven health product or one with audacious claims, check with your health care professional first (www.ftc.gov).

19. Which Supplements are most effective?

Keep in mind that the Food and Drug Administration (FDA) does not evaluate dietary supplements' effectiveness, safety, or quality of their ingredients before they enter the marketplace. Therefore, there is no guarantee that the product contains what it says it does. Furthermore, a product may even have varying ingredients from batch to batch.

FDA does require supplement manufacturers to adhere to Current Good Manufacturing Practices (CGMP) to ensure the quality and safety of their products, but compliance is not always enforced. To ensure the quality of a product, look for one certified by a third-party company. Third-party testing is not required by law, however, some supplement manufacturers voluntarily undergo testing to show their commitment to producing high-quality supplements.

The Certificate of Analysis (COA) is an objective indicator of product quality granted by an independent third-party company, such as USP, NSF, Banned Substances Control Group (BSCG), or ConsumerLab. These third-party companies will test for one or more of the following :

a. The supplement contains what's stated on the label and in the amounts listed.

b. Products are standardized from batch to batch.

c. The supplement is free of harmful contaminants or other potential drug contaminants.

d. The product doesn't contain any undeclared ingredients.

e. Also, if you're an athlete, look for National Sanitation Foundation (NSF) Certified for Sport products. The certification ensures that the product is free of over 270 substances banned or prohibited by most major sports organizations.

20. Does it Matter what Brand of Supplements you Buy?

Many companies use multibranding to sell the same product under different labels and markets to appeal to different market segments or categories. You may walk into a store and see multiple competing brands on the same shelf made by the same supplier. For example, companies like Trader Joe's or Costco don't make their vitamins. They have a reputable source that makes them for them who is also selling under their brand somewhere else and probably making vitamins for other companies.

Because vitamins and minerals are commodity items, most manufacturers have access to the same ingredients. When scientists measure vitamins in the blood, they find the same levels whether they take a generic brand or a name brand. For that reason, paying more for a name brand won't necessarily buy you better supplements. Pick a reputable source such as Costco's Kirkland brand, which is likely to use the best suppliers to avoid tarnishing their brand due to poor quality products and frequently restocking fresh product due to brisk business. Larger retailers such as Costco also strive only to sell products that provide dosages of crucial ingredients high enough to impact your health to maintain a loyal customer base. For example, CoQ10, a relatively well-tolerated and safe supplement, can be bought inexpensively at low dosages of 10 mg soft gels. However, 90–200 mg of CoQ10 per day is recommended, and some conditions require higher dosages of 300–600 mg. Costco only sells the 300 mg soft gel, which is ideal for most people. Costco doesn't waste shelf space selling multiple options of the same item. They typically only offer the perfect product in its category, making the buying process much more manageable.

Remember that price does not assure quality. The product label is what is the most important. If you consider a vitamin supplement, read the label and compare the information and ingredients. Some vitamins contain more fillers than the actual active ingredient. You also want to make sure the supplement is geared towards your sex, age group, and lifestyle.

Examine the label, check for active ingredients, nutrients included, and the serving size, such as a capsule or packet, as well as the number of nutrients in that particular serving. Avoid megadosing on supplements, the general rule of thumb is to choose a vitamin supplement that provides 100 percent of the Daily Value unless you have a specific identified need for more of a particular supplement.

21. Can I take expired Supplements?

Expired supplements are not necessarily unsafe to consume. However, the supplement's potency decreases the older the supplement gets and eventually becomes inactive. It is best to discard that product and purchase a new batch. Keep track of expiration dates.

22. Can I Cut Supplements in Half if I have difficulty swallowing them?

Most tablets can be crushed or cut up as long as you're still consuming the entire pill. Softgels can be punctured and released into a spoon or food source. The gel coating should also be consumed as they sometimes have supplement ingredients. The only exceptions are time-release or enteric-coated supplements. Other options are gummies, chewable vitamins, or powder supplements as alternatives to tablets.

23. What are good Resources for Picking Supplements?

Databases

Dietary Supplement Ingredient Database (DSID)

The DSID provides estimated levels of ingredients in dietary supplement products sold in the United States. The DSID was developed by the Methods and Application of Food Composition Laboratory in collaboration with the Office of Dietary Supplements at the National Institutes of Health (NIH) and other federal agencies. DSID-4 reports national estimates of ingredient content in adult, children's, and non-prescription prenatal multivitamin/mineral (MVMs) and omega-3 fatty acid supplements. The DSID is intended primarily for research applications. These data are appropriate for use in population studies of nutrient intake rather than for assessing the content of individual products.

Dietary Supplement Label Database (DSLD)

The DSLD from the Office of Dietary Supplements (ODS) at the National Institutes of Health (NIH) provides information taken from the labels of dietary supplement products sold in the United States. This information includes the name and form of the ingredients, amounts of the nutritional components and percent of the Daily Value (DV) of nutrients, the manufacturer/distributor, health-related claims, warning statements, and an image of the package label. In June 2013, the DSLD began as a resource for researchers, health care providers, and consumers.

Computer Access to Research on Dietary Supplements (CARDS) Database

CARDS is a database of federally funded research projects on dietary supplements. Currently, CARDS contains projects financed by the United States Department of Agriculture (USDA), the Department of Defense (DOD), and the Institutes and Centers (I.C.s) of the National Institutes of Health (NIH) beginning the fiscal year 1999.

PubMed

PubMed is a search engine specialized in biomedical and life sciences literature to improve health globally and personally. PubMed was developed in 1996 and has been maintained by the National Center for Biotechnology Information (NCBI) in the U.S. National Library of Medicine (NLM), located at the National Institutes of Health (NIH). The database contains more than 32 million citations and abstracts of biomedical literature. It does not include full-text journal articles; however, links to the full text are often present when available from other sources, such as the publisher's website or PubMed Central (PMC).

ClinicalTrials.gov

ClinicalTrials.gov is a web-based resource that provides patients, their family members, health care professionals, researchers, and the public with easy access to publicly and privately supported clinical studies on a wide range of diseases and conditions. The website is maintained by the National Library of Medicine (NLM) at the National Institutes of Health (NIH).

NIH RePORT
The Research Portfolio Online Reporting Tools (RePORT) provide access to reports, data, and analyses of NIH research activities, including information on NIH expenditures and the results of NIH-supported research.

USDA Databases
Food and nutrient databases from the U.S. Department of Agriculture, including data sets for pro-anthocyanidins, flavonoids, choline, iodine, fluoride, isoflavones, and glucosinolates.

USDA FoodData
The U.S. Department of Agriculture FoodData website provides detailed information on the nutrient content of foods consumed in the U.S., including a subset of American Indian/Alaska Native Foods.

Consumerlab.com
Consumer lab is a publisher of test results on health, wellness, and nutrition products. Consumer Labs is not a laboratory but contracts studies to outside laboratories.

The U.S. Pharmocopoeia (USP)
USP is an independent, scientific nonprofit organization focused on building trust in the supply of safe, quality medicines. They strengthen the global supply chain so that drugs people rely on for health are available when needed and work as expected (www.ods.od.nih.gov).

24. What Vitamin Combinations Should You Avoid?

I thought my vitamin might be cancerous. Fortunately, the tests showed it was B-9.

Magnesium and Calcium/Multivitamin
Taking magnesium and a multivitamin simultaneously can interfere with the absorption of smaller minerals found in the multivitamin, like iron and zinc.

Also, don't take calcium, magnesium, or zinc together as they will compete for absorption. For best results, take them two hours apart.

Vitamins E, and K

Vitamin E supplementation can increase bleeding in some people. Some doctors prescribe a vitamin K supplement to help with blood clotting to prevent this. Taking vitamin E with vitamin K can counteract the effects of vitamin K.

Fish Oil & Ginkgo Biloba

Both have blood-thinning potentials, and taking both together can increase the risk for uncontrollable bleeding or inability to clot.

Copper and Zinc

Zinc boosts the immune system and promotes healing but can interfere with your body's absorption of copper. Some minerals compete for absorption in your digestive system when taken simultaneously. For example, if you take copper and zinc together, copper will be poorly absorbed, and zinc wins. People sometimes develop a copper deficiency when they take a lot of zinc. If you take copper supplements because of copper deficiency, avoid taking zinc simultaneously. If you must take both, take them at least two hours apart.

Denture creams are a source of zinc supplementation. If you use denture cream and experience neurological problems, you may have a copper deficiency.

Iron and Green Tea

Individually, both of these supplements offer a lot of benefits. Iron is essential for making a hemoglobin protein that carries oxygen in your blood. Green tea has anti-inflammatory compounds that help people with conditions like inflammatory bowel disease.

Green tea can cause iron deficiency if taken in large quantities for more extended periods. On the other hand, iron can decrease the efficacy of green tea. The antioxidants in green tea can bind to and neutralize the effects of iron when taken together. Skip green tea on days when you're taking your iron supplement.

Vitamin C and B12

Vitamin C can reduce B12 absorption by breaking it down in your digestive tract. Because of this, wait at least two hours before taking Vitamin C with your Vitamin B12.

Vitamin A Supplements and Vitamin A-rich Foods

Since vitamin A is a fat-soluble vitamin, any excess is stored in body fat. So, we don't need to take vitamin A every day. Too much vitamin A can weaken your bones and lead to more bone fractures as you age.

Excess vitamin A can also be harmful to unborn babies. Avoid eating liver or liver paté if you're pregnant or take a vitamin A supplement. These foods are so high in vitamin A that you should only eat them once a week to avoid consuming too much, even if you do not take a vitamin A supplement.

Folic Acid (Vitamin B9) and Vitamin B12

While both B vitamins are essential, taking too much folic acid or folate can hide vitamin B12 deficiency symptoms. So, have your blood levels checked before adding these supplements to your regimen.

Table 1
Drug Interactions with Vitamins and Minerals

Vitamin/Mineral Supplement	Affected Medication	Effect of Interaction	Management of Interaction
Vitamin A	Retinoids (isotretinoin and acitretin)	Risk of toxicity; nausea, vomiting, dizziness, blurred vision, poor muscle coordination	Avoid concomitant use
Pyridoxine (Vitamin B_6)	Levodopa	Decreased efficacy leading to parkinsonian symptoms	Recommend carbidopa/levodopa combination
	Phenytoin	Risk of seizure	Discontinue pyridoxine or increase phenytoin dose
Vitamin E	Warfarin	Risk of bleeding	Avoid doses ≥800 IU/day of vitamin E
Vitamin K	Warfarin	Decreased efficacy; risk of thromboembolism	Maintain consistent intake of vitamin K
Niacin	HMG-CoA reductase inhibitors	Risk of myopathy or rhabdomyolysis	Avoid self-treatment with niacin
Folic acid	Methotrexate	Prevents adverse events or toxicities from methotrexate	Recommend supplementation in patients taking methotrexate for rheumatoid arthritis or psoriasis
Calcium	Fluoroquinolones and tetracyclines	Decreased efficacy; risk of antibiotic failure	Avoid concomitant calcium supplementation
	Levothyroxine and bisphosphonates	Decreased efficacy; risk of hypothyroidism	Separate doses by at least four hours
Aluminum and magnesium	Fluoroquinolones, tetracyclines, bisphosphonates, and levothyroxine	Decreased efficacy of affected medication	Separate doses by at least two hours
Iron	Fluoroquinolones, tetracyclines, digoxin, and levothyroxine	Decreased efficacy of affected medication	Separate doses by at least two hours
	Methyldopa	Worsening of hypertension	Avoid concomitant use
Potassium (including salt substitutes)	ACE inhibitors, angiotensin receptor blockers, digoxin, indomethacin, prescription potassium supplements, and potassium-sparing diuretics	Hyperkalemia	Avoid concomitant supplementation without physician supervision

ACE: angiotensin-converting enzyme.

Many drugs interact with vitamins, herbal products, and minerals, ranging in severity and significance. Often patients may not think to share information with their healthcare provider or feel the substances are harmless and irrelevant to their medication regimen. Because of the possibility of drug interaction, consumers should be upfront about the supplements they take so their healthcare providers can educate them about possible reactions and allergies. Healthcare providers cannot provide the necessary screening for interactions without this information.

25. Do vitamins and minerals make up for a poor diet?

My doctor was making fun of me for being low on B vitamins...

He's giving me a complex.

Whole foods provide perfectly balanced nutrients that our bodies have evolved to absorb. Nutrient-dense foods contain essential vitamins and minerals, dietary fiber, and other naturally occurring substances that support good health. The goal should always be to meet your nutritional needs through healthy eating.

Dietary supplements can never replace the benefits of a healthy diet because they are not a complete source of nutrients such as fresh fruits, vegetables, whole grains, eggs, some animal proteins, and high-quality fats.

26. Who needs to take supplements?

Most people can get all their nutrient needs met from a nutrient-dense diet. However, most people don't, and there are specific situations where a dietary supplement may benefit.

a. Pregnant women should take a folic acid supplement, consume foods fortified with folic acid, or both during childbearing years. The probability of specific congenital disabilities, which can occur before pregnancy, can be reduced. Look for prenatal vitamins that contain methyl folate, a form of folate that is easier to absorb.

b. Adolescent girls and pregnant women are at risk for iron-deficiency anemia. A blood test can diagnose this condition, reversible with dietary changes or an iron supplement.

c. People with liver disease, cystic fibrosis, celiac disease, Crohn's disease, obesity, gastric bypass, seniors, breastfed infants, people in northern hemispheres, and dark skin may need extra vitamin D.

d. People who have food allergies, a medical condition, or a vegan diet benefit from a multivitamin/multimineral. For example, vegans need to supplement vitamin B12 because animal foods are the primary dietary source of this essential nutrient.

Seniors also have more difficulty absorbing vitamin B12 and vitamin D as they age.

e. Individuals who eat low-calorie or restrictive diets because of poor appetite, drug and alcohol abuse, or an eating disorder will need supplements to reduce the risk of nutrient deficiencies and malnutrition. For example Iron helps transport oxygen in the blood. Not enough iron may result in a weak immune system and fatigue. Men and women should consume between 8 to 18 milligrams of iron daily. Iron is found in red meats, leafy green vegetables, and legumes. However, plant-based sources of iron don't absorb as well because the amount of fiber in a vegetarian or vegan diet can block iron. So vegetarians and vegans are at risk for iron deficiency and should supplement.

f. Bariatric surgery can impair your ability to absorb nutrients, increasing the risk of nutrient deficiencies. Therefore a post surgery protocol almost always includes a supplement regime.

27. How are vitamins and supplements regulated?

The Food and Drug Administration (FDA) is the federal agency responsible for assessing the safety of dietary supplements after they reach the market. The FDA monitors health claims on product packaging, keeps track of side effects reported by consumers and health care providers, and performs safety research. If a product is misrepresented or unsafe, the FDA can issue a warning to the manufacturer or require it to be removed from the marketplace.

Supplements are not always harmless because they are "natural." Some supplements are adulterated with pharmaceuticals or closely related compounds, including stimulants, bodybuilding steroids, antidepressants, weight loss medications, and drugs to treat erectile dysfunction, all with sometimes dangerous side effects.

28. What to consider when choosing supplements?

Over 20,000 visits to the ER a year are due to dietary supplements. Some supplements have side effects, interact with medications, or are not tolerated by some people.

a. Most dietary supplements have not been tested on pregnant and nursing women, infants, or children.

b. Discuss supplementation with your healthcare provider and always follow the directions on the label for the correct dosage.

29. How can I evaluate the quality of a supplement?

Do some research using credible sources such as;

a. The National Center for Complementary and Integrative Health (NCCIH) and the National Institutes of Health's (NIH) Office of Dietary Supplements (ODS) is a reliable source of free information. The NIH has created MedlinePlus, a health information website that offers information about dietary supplements' effectiveness, usual dosage, and drug interactions.

b. The Natural Medicines Comprehensive Database current facts and ratings on the effectiveness and safety of over 1100 natural medicines.

c. The United States Pharmacopeia (USP) and National Science Foundation (NSF) are independent, nongovernmental organizations that evaluate supplements. They don't verify the effectiveness of a product, but they do confirm the identity, strength, and purity of supplements.

d. ConsumerLab is a private publisher of reviews and independent test results on wellness, health, and nutrition products.

30. What supplements should I consider?

Many nutrients work synergistically to allow the body to function optimally. So, how do you know which ones to take?

Our individual nutrient needs can vary as much as a fingerprint does. Your nutrient profile can be affected by your genes, microbiome (bacteria in your body that make up 10% of your body weight), diet, lifestyle, culture, race, pharmaceutical drugs, environment, weather, and gender. For this reason, it's best to get a blood test at your doctor's office to determine your nutrient levels and possible vitamin deficiencies. Periodic testing will help you identify potential deficits and what supplements and dosage may be needed. Below is a list of the recommended daily allowance (RDA), recommended amounts, foods rich in each vitamin, and how to get them through supplements if you're not getting them.

VITAMINS

Vitamin	RDA Men	RDA Women	Best Sources	Functions
A (carotene)	900ug	700ug	Yellow or orange fruits and vegetables, green leafy vegetables, liver, dairy products	Formation and maintenance of skin, hair and mucous membranes, helps you see in dim light, bone and tooth growth
B1 (thiamine)	1.2 mg	1.1 mg	Fortified cereals and oatmeal, meats, rice and pasta, whole grains, liver	Helps body release energy from carbohydrates during metabolism, growth and muscle tone
B2 (riboflavin)	1.3 mg	1.1 mg	Whole grains, green leafy vegetables, organ meats, milk, eggs	Helps body release energy from protein, fat and carbohydrates, during metabolism
B6 (pyridoxine)	1.3 mg	1.3 mg	Fish, poultry, lean meats, bananas, prunes, dried beans, whole grains, avocados	Helps build tissues and aids in metabolism of protein
B12 (cobalamin)	2.4ug	2.4ug	Meats, milk products, seafood	Aids cell development, functioning of nervous system and metabolism of fat and protein
Biotin	30ug	30ug	Cereal/grain products, yeast, legumes, liver	Involved in metabolism of protein, fats, carbohydrates
Choline	550 mg	425 mg	Milk, liver, eggs, peanuts	A precursor acetylcholine, essential for liver function
Folate (folic acid, folacin)	400ug	400ug	Green leafy vegetables, organ meats, dried peas, beans, lentils	Aids in genetic material development, red cell production
Niacin	16 mg	14 mg	Meat, poultry, fish, enriched cereals, peanuts, potatoes, dairy products, eggs	Involved in carbohydrate, protein and fat metabolism
Pantothenic Acid	5 mg	5 mg	Lean meats, whole grains, legumes, vegetables, fruits	Helps release energy from fats and carbohydrates
C (ascorbic acid)	90 mg	75 mg	Citrus fruits, berries, vegetables-especially peppers	Essential for structure of bones and cartilage, muscle and blood vessels, helps maintain capillaries and gums and aids in absorption of iron.
D	5ug	5ug	Fortified milk, sunlight, fish, eggs, butter	Aids in bone and tooth formation; helps maintain heart action and nervous system
E	15 mg	15 mg	Fortified and multigrain cereals, nuts, wheat germ, vegetable oils, green leafy vegetables	Protects blood cells, body tissue, and essential fatty acids from harmful destruction
K	120ug	90ug	Green leafy vegetables, fruit, dairy products and grains	Essential for blood clotting functions

31. How long do supplements stay in my system?

Nutraceuticals (food or supplements that contain health-benefiting additives) differ significantly in the amount of time the active ingredient(s) remain in your body. Fat-soluble nutrients, like vitamin A, can be stored in the liver for weeks and released to body tissues as needed. Water-soluble nutrients, such as vitamin C, will generally be metabolized and leave the body the same day of use or even within a few hours after consumption.

32. How long should I take a supplement before deciding if it works or not?

The observation period depends on the supplement and the expected outcome. For example, melatonin generally works within the first week or even the first day. On the other hand, joint-health ingredients glucosamine and chondroitin usually take six to eight weeks before working.

33. Is it OK to take a supplement one day but not the next?

It depends on the supplement. For example, vitamin D is stored in fat cells, so you don't have to take it every day because your body can release it from body fat stores when needed. However, maintenance supplements, such as multivitamins, ginseng, or chlorella, should be taken daily, as should any supplement taken for long-term therapeutic effects. Then some supplements can be used acutely for specific results, and those don't have to be taken daily. Valerian root, for example, is taken for better sleep or L-theanine taken for stress relief generally does not need to be taken daily but can be used situationally.

34. What is the best supplement form?

There are a wide variety of options available for supplement delivery systems. Popularized by the pharmaceutical industry, common pill forms include tablets, hard capsules, and soft capsules. Other supplements take the form of lozenges, liquids, powders, gels, gummy vitamins, and even vitamin injections.

Deciding on what form to take a supplement depends on the active ingredient and the consumer. Children, for example, are much happier eating a chewable, gel, or gummy vitamin. However, these kid-friendly forms have drawbacks compared to swallowed tablets or capsules and require special handling. In contrast, they might struggle to swallow tablets.

Tablets and Capsules

Well-made tablets or capsules are the most effective delivery system, making it the most used form of most pharmaceutical medications. Years of controlled clinical studies have confirmed that they're a reliable, efficient drug delivery system.

These products can also provide more active ingredients (much more than a liquid, gel, or gummy). Because they require fewer excipients, which is an ingredient that does not serve a functional nutritional purpose. They're included for stability, digestibility, manufacturing, or similar purposes. The shelf-life and stability of tablets are also superior to gummy or liquid vitamins.

Vitamin, mineral, and antioxidant supplements that do not need hefty (> 2 grams) doses are best taken in tablet and capsule form. For example, vitamin C, B vitamins, iron, or iodine all have typical daily amounts small enough to be included easily. Many of these nutrients also have a bad taste that can be easily hidden in this form and not in other states.

Tablet and Capsule Pros:
Hides bad tastes
Long shelf-life
Concentrated delivery of active ingredients (fewer excipients)
Tablet and Capsule Cons:
Not appropriate for sizeable active ingredient doses
Difficult for some to swallow

Chewable Tablets

Chewables are the best supplement for people who have trouble swallowing whole capsules or tablets. Like other tablets, chewable has a long shelf life and is best used for ingredients only in smaller (< 2 grams) doses.

Tablets are usually chewable, so bad-tasting elements can be masked with sweeteners and flavorings. This can become a limitation as some sugar can be used. Some chewable multivitamin, multi-mineral products also do not have essential minerals such as selenium, chromium, magnesium, or zinc because it is hard to hide their flavors.

Chewable Tablet Pros:
Long shelf-life
Easy to consume

Chewable Tablet Cons:
Added sweeteners (although typically minimal amounts)
Not as concentrated as swallowed tablets
May be missing key ingredients

Gummy Vitamins

Gummy vitamins, similar to chewable tablets, are better tasting for children and those who have trouble swallowing tablets. However, gummy vitamins can be over-consumed like candy, causing dosage beyond the recommended amount due to their taste. Gummies are also even more limited than chewable tablets in what ingredients they can contain. Gummies often have very few or are absent of essential minerals and contain much smaller doses of the ingredients they do possess. Gummies are best used for supplements that only need to be taken in minimal amounts (< 100mg).

Gummy Pros:
Great tasting
Easy to consume

Gummy Cons:
Added sweeteners
Not compatible with many ingredients

Powders

Powders can include larger doses (> 2 grams) of some nutrients and are easy to consume. The active ingredients in powdered supplements can be tasted, so they must be palatable or easily masked. They must also contain soluble ingredients that can be shaken up in the liquid.

Protein powder is the most popular powdered supplement. Because it requires doses too large for a tablet or capsule, it is ideal for this form of delivery. It is also easy to make taste good and mixes easily with water. Other ingredients such as branched-chain amino acids (BCAAs), creatine, caffeine, or immune-boosting formulas are commonly found in powders and quickly mix with water.

Powder Pros:
Can include large doses of active ingredients
Inexpensive to transport

Powder Cons:
Added sweeteners and excipients
Less concentrated active ingredients (more excipients)

Liquids
Liquid supplements are similar to powders, except they're already mixed with a liquid. They generally have powdered supplements' same ingredients, benefits, and drawbacks.

Liquid supplements are best for powders such as protein, branched-chain amino acids (BCAAs), creatine, and caffeine. They can also include micronutrients such as vitamins and minerals and other antioxidants.

Liquid supplements have a shorter shelf-life than their powdered equivalent because they're already mixed. Liquid supplements may also require "other" ingredients, such as emulsifiers, solvents, preservatives, stabilizing agents, coloring, and flavoring.

Liquids Pros:
Can include large doses of active ingredients
More convenient than mixing powders

Liquids Cons:
Difficult to add non-soluble ingredients
More expensive and difficult to transport
Less concentrated active ingredients (more excipients)
Often a shorter shelf-life
Added sweeteners and excipients

Vitamin Injections
Injections are great for delivering select nutrients in large doses. Specific vitamins can be injected intravenously (IV) or by intramuscular injections. Vitamin B12 and C are more effective when injected in some populations. However, because of the

possibilities of infection, bleeding (hematoma), or embolism, injections should only be given under a healthcare professional's recommendation.

Vitamin Injection Pros:
Can deliver high doses of select nutrients

Vitamin Injection Cons:
Uncomfortable
Limited nutrient compatibility
Potential health risks

35. What is the Best Supplement Form?

Consider your needs, what you're comfortable with, and what your healthcare professionals recommend. Consider the pros and cons of each, depending on your needs. The essential factor to keep in mind is what you need to do to be compliant with your supplement regime. Some people make a sizable investment in supplements but don't use them because they don't like swallowing pills. So make sure that you're getting something that you're comfortable using to be compliant.

36. What's the difference between the RDA, DRI, and DV for a vitamin or mineral?

They are all the same, and there is no difference. The Recommended Daily Allowance (RDA), Daily Value (DV), and the Dietary Reference Intake (DRI) all mean the same thing. They were established in 1943 as a guide for planning and procuring food supplies for national defense. They state the minimum amount of nutrients the general population needs to stave off a deficiency disease. For example, most healthy people need 90 mg of vitamin C per day to avoid scurvy.

37. How much should I be taking?

Take the recommended intake levels of essential nutrients. Read the labels of the supplements you're considering to find a supplement formula in these ranges. Be mindful that you may have to take multiple supplements as you will not find a formula that provides these nutrients at the recommended levels in one pill. It would be too big. For example, many one-a-day supplements offer good levels of vitamins, but they're insufficient in minerals. Our bodies need the minerals just as much as it requires the vitamins. The two work together.

Here are optimum intake ranges of vitamins:

Age	11 – 14	15 – 18	19 – 24	25 – 50	+51
Calories (kCal)	2500	3000	2900	2900	3000
Protein (g)	45	59	58	63	63
Vitamin A (ug)	1000	1000	1000	1000	1000
Vitamin D (ug)	10	10	10	5	5
Vitamin E (mg)	10	10	10	10	10
Vitamin K (ug)	45	65	70	80	80
Vitamin C (mg)	50	60	60	60	60
Thiamin (mg)	1.3	1.5	1.5	1.5	1.2
Riboflavin (mg)	1.5	1.8	1.7	1.7	1.4
Niacin (mg)	17	20	19	19	15
Vitamin B6 (ug)	1.7	2	2	2	2
Folate (ug)	150	200	200	200	200
Vitamin B12 (mg)	2.0	2.0	2.0	2.0	2.0
Calcium (mg)	1200	1200	1200	800	800
Phosphorous (mg)	1200	1200	1200	800	800
Magnesium (mg)	270	400	350	350	350
Iron (mg)	12	12	10	10	10
Zinc (ug)	15	15 – 18	15	15	15
Iodine (ug)	150	150	150	150	150
Selenium (ug)	40	50	70	70	70

38. Can I be healthy without taking supplements?

The idea of optimal health is what drives people to take nutritional supplements. There is a big difference between the minimum amount of a nutrient required to avoid getting sick and the maximum for optimal function. There's more to living in a state of vitality than just not being sick.

39. Are probiotics something I should take long-term or only immediately after taking an antibiotic?

If you eat the recommended amount of fruits and vegetables every day, probiotics are unnecessary. However, most people do not eat the recommended amounts, so everyone (except those immunocompromised) can and should consume them every day. More probiotics are being recommended simply as part of a healthful diet. Make sure you take prebiotics to feed the probiotics.

40. Can supplements interact with prescribed medications?

Yes, some of them can. For example, St. John's wort is often taken for mild depression, but it can increase the metabolism of or reduce the blood concentrations of several prescribed drugs.

It may increase the metabolism of oral contraceptive estrogens, decrease the effects of Xanax, prolong narcotic-induced sleep time, and change the effects of some antihypertensive drugs. Most other medicinal herbs, including echinacea, garlic, ginkgo, ginseng, goldenseal, and milk thistle, don't regularly interfere with prescribed medications; in 2012, German researchers concluded these six botanicals produce no adverse effects when interacting with pharmaceuticals. Inversely some prescribed drugs can interfere with or deplete the body with some essential nutrients. For example, statins, which are taken to lower cholesterol levels, can deplete the body of coenzyme Q10.

41. Can I trust the health claims made on a supplement box?

Claims on supplements can be easily misinterpreted. Supplements are regulated as foods, not as pharmaceutical drugs. The FDA says only drugs can treat diseases. As a result, a supplement can't legally claim to treat a disease, such as diabetes or heart disease. Supplements have their class of claims called "structure and function" claims. Meaning that a supplement maker is only allowed to communicate a possible health effect on the structure of an organ or the function of a part of the body's physiology. Therefore a bottle of glucosamine and chondroitin won't say, "This joint-health formula cures arthritic pain," but it could say something like, "This formula supports joint health." Even though research shows a joint-health formula can cure joint pain in some cases, the manufacturer can't specifically say that according to the law.

42. Should I buy synthetic or organic supplements?

Organic supplements, also called natural supplements, are derived from real food, while synthetic supplements are made in a lab. Some people prefer organic supplements because they are made from whole foods. However, no matter where the supplement comes from, your body uses it the same.

Benefits of organic versus synthetic

Synthetic vitamins are less expensive than the organic kind. Also, many natural vitamins require taking multiple doses a day, which can be easier to tolerate when taken in smaller amounts throughout the day. In the end, both organic and synthetic vitamins will give you the desired outcomes.

43. Does taking vitamins make you gain weight?

No, vitamins cannot directly increase your weight, as they hardly have any calories. However, vitamin deficiencies can lead to adverse weight effects.

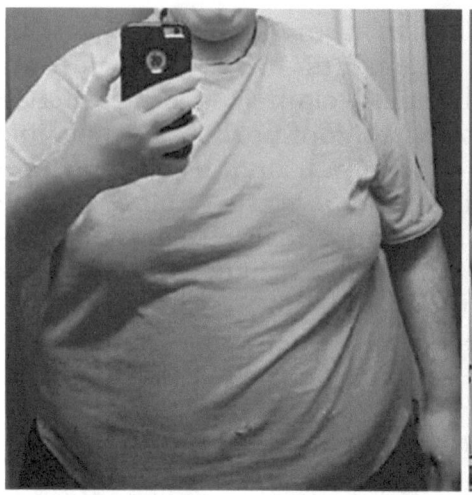
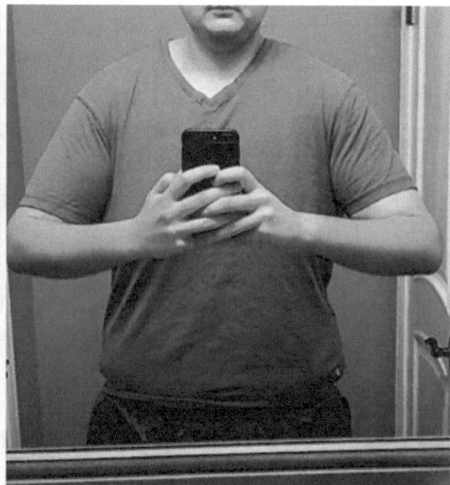

One of the most common health issues encountered by people deficient in nutrients is obesity. Rick was a patient that was 6' 4", 420 lbs. he reminded me of an offensive lineman for the National Football League. However, Rick did not want to be an American football player, he wanted a girlfriend, and he felt that his weight was the number one obstacle to meeting the ideal woman. He tried countless diets and exercise regimens with little success. I decided to test his vitamin D levels. The typical vitamin D range is between 20 and 40 nanograms per milliliter (ng/mL). Rick's vitamin D level was 8 ng/mL. Rick described his daily routine as being indoors throughout the day and only coming out at night to do shopping or errands. Rick also worked at night and slept during the day, so his exposure to natural sunlight was minimal. He estimated his daily sunlight exposure was 5 minutes a day on a good day. Experts believe that if you don't get at least 30 minutes a day of sunlight, it does the same damage to your health as smoking a pack of cigarettes.

The solution was for Rick to sit outside for at least 30 minutes a day while he ate his lunch and start a vitamin D regimen to get his vitamin D levels up. Rick quickly started shedding 2 lbs. a week over two months without changing his diet or exercising. Once he lost 16 lbs. he became motivated and started dieting and exercising, resulting in much more weight loss getting him closer to his ideal weight.

44. Which vitamins are best taken together?

1. Iron + Vitamin C

Taking iron and vitamin C together helps boost iron absorption.

2. Vitamin D + Calcium

Both nutrients are essential for bone health. Calcium will get absorbed on its own, but if you eat smaller amounts, vitamin D can help the intestines absorb Calcium. It may also help with the absorption of phosphorous, another bone-building mineral.

3. Vitamin B12 + Folate (B9)

Vitamin B12 and folate work together in the body for cell division and replication. Folate is a B vitamin, and it depends on vitamin B12 to be absorbed, stored, and used by the body.

4. Potassium + sodium

Potassium and sodium are electrolytes that help your body maintain fluid and blood volume to function normally. However, consuming too little potassium and too much sodium can raise your blood pressure. Though "salt" and "sodium" are used interchangeably, they do not mean the same thing.

5. Vitamin D + Omega-3s

Vitamin D is a fat-soluble vitamin, meaning that it needs fat to be absorbed. Omega-3 supplements can help the body absorb vitamin D.

6. Magnesium + Vitamin D

Magnesium is a critical factor in making Vitamin D bioavailable. Vitamin D is stored in the body and can not be used without the presence of magnesium. The body depends on magnesium to convert Vitamin D into its active form within the body. However its best to take vitamin D in the mornings otherwise it'll disrupt the production of melatonin and disturb your sleep. While magnesium is best at night so it promotes better sleep.

7. Vitamin D + Vitamin K

Vitamins D and K should be taken together. They help the body use calcium ideally for building bone instead of depositing it dangerously in arteries and soft tissue.

45. Which vitamins should not be taken together?

1. Zinc + Copper + Phosphorus + Iron

It is best to space zinc, copper, iron, and phosphorus supplements 2 hours apart to get the full benefit from each dietary supplement.

2. Iron + Calcium

Calcium can inhibit the absorption of iron in both food and supplement forms.

46. Should I take supplements with food?

Most supplements are absorbed better when taken with food to reduce the chances of upsetting your stomach and stimulating absorption by slowing down the transit time through the GI tract.

When taken on an empty stomach, iron, magnesium, and fish oil supplements are most likely to upset your stomach, so take these with food.

Fat-soluble vitamins A, D, E, and K are better absorbed when taken with at least a teaspoon of fat (around 5 grams of fat). For example, when taking your multivitamin, have some almond butter with your oatmeal or butter with your toast.

Researchers suggest taking probiotics with a meal or 30 minutes before a meal instead of after eating.

Fluid intake is crucial for the disintegration of the supplement tablet or capsule, and the dissolution of water-soluble nutrients such as B vitamins and C. Drink a large glass of water with all of your supplements.

The only supplements that should be taken without food are chelated minerals. Chelation occurs when a mineral is bound to acid, so it doesn't rely on your stomach acid to break it down. Calcium citrate and magnesium glycinate are the primary examples.

Best with Food
CoQ10*
Fat-Soluble Vitamins A, D, E, and K*
Fish Oil/Omega-3*
Multivitamin*
Prenatal Multivitamin*

Magnesium
Vitamin C
* Consume at least one teaspoon, or about 5 grams, of fat to maximize absorption.

Okay without Food
Chelated Mineral Supplements (i.e., magnesium glycinate and calcium citrate) Chelated minerals can be taken on an empty stomach because they do not need stomach acid to break them down.

Iron
Iron is absorbed better on an empty stomach, however, it causes GI upset for some. If iron upsets your stomach, take it with a meal to reduce GI upset.

Better Together
Vitamin D, Calcium, Vitamin K2, and Magnesium
Vitamin C and Iron

Better Apart
Calcium
When taking a separate calcium supplement >200mg per dose, take it 1-2 hours apart from multivitamins or supplements containing iron, zinc, magnesium, folate, or fiber.

If your multivitamin contains calcium, as long as it is <200mg per dose, it should not interfere with the absorption of other nutrients.

Magnesium
When taking a separate magnesium supplement >250mg per dose, take it 1-2 hours apart from multivitamins or supplements containing iron, zinc, calcium, folate, or fiber.

Zinc
Zinc can interfere with your body's absorption of copper. If you must take both, take them at least two hours apart.

47. Five factors that can Interfere with Nutrient Absorption

A. Alcohol: Alcohol affects the absorption of nutrients by causing the quick breakdown of capsules and pills before they reach the small intestine where absorption happens. It can also prevent normal digestion by damaging cells in the stomach and intestine and interfering with the release of digestive enzymes. Alcohol is also a diuretic, promoting the excretion of stored minerals such as magnesium and calcium. You can prevent alcohol's negative impact on nutrient absorption by avoiding it within four hours of taking supplements.

 B. Caffeine: Like alcohol, caffeine can cause the excretion of minerals and vitamins. Excessive amounts of tannins (a type of plant compound) found in caffeine can inhibit the absorption of B-vitamins, calcium, iron, and magnesium. Drink decaffeinated beverages or reduce the consumption of coffee or tea to 1 or 2 per day between meals.

 C. Prescription drugs: Some medications can bind with nutrients and prevent absorption. For example, acid-reducing drugs can decrease the absorption of vitamin B12, and antibiotics can destroy "good" bacteria in the digestive system that help with the digestion and absorption of vitamins and minerals. Inversely some supplements can interfere with the effectiveness of medications. Therefore it's recommended to consult with a healthcare professional to discuss possible interactions and ensure you're obtaining and absorbing essential nutrients.

 D. Stress: Uncontrolled stress can deplete your body of nutrient stores and alter your body's digestive efficiency. If you're feeling stressed, make sure you're getting enough antioxidants (including vitamins A, C, and E), fiber, B-vitamins, and minerals such as chromium, copper, iron, magnesium, and zinc as the uptake of these nutrients can decrease during times of stress.

 E. Age: Your body becomes less efficient at extracting and absorbing nutrients from the foods you eat and the supplements you take as you age. Eating a nutrient-dense whole food diet, primarily fruits, and vegetables, will help. Have your vitamin levels tested regularly, so you can address any specific deficiencies.

48. Why do multivitamins have vitamins and minerals that counteract? Are multivitamins good?

 Most multivitamins are formulated in such a way as to counteract any potential negative nutrient-nutrient interactions. They contain the appropriate levels of synergistic and antagonistic nutrients, meaning that some vitamins and minerals can enhance or inhibit others.

For example, magnesium can increase vitamin D levels. Yet, vitamin A can decrease vitamin D uptake. For this reason, you'll almost always find the percentage daily value (% DV) of vitamin D is higher than vitamin A on most multivitamin nutrition labels. The downside is that you could be getting too much or too little of a particular vitamin or mineral. If you're deficient in vitamin A, taking a multivitamin might not fill your nutritional need. Inversely, excess fat-soluble vitamins A, D, E, and K from food and/or supplements can build up in your body and become toxic, causing severe health problems.

Another issue with multivitamins is the limited space inside them. Some essential nutrients are either not included or in minimal amounts (≤ 250 mg): i.e., calcium and magnesium. They are considered macronutrients because we need to obtain them in large quantities. The daily calcium requirements for men and women aged 51-70 years are 1,000 mg and 1,200 mg, respectively. For men and women of the same age group, the daily requirements for magnesium are 420 mg and 320 mg, respectively. (Compare these recommended intake values with those of the micronutrient selenium, which is 55 mcg for men and women aged ≥ 51 years.). So calcium and magnesium are included in small doses to allow space for other nutrients and avoid competing with other nutrients for absorption in the body.

Multivitamins are suitable for people who simply don't want to take supplements and know they won't have any interactions with any of the ingredients because of a specific health disorder. At the very least, it gives you some of the essential nutrients you need to thrive. However, single vitamin or mineral supplements tailored to support individual health goals or address nutrient deficiencies may are preferred over multivitamins.

Look for a multivitamin that has less or none of these conflicting ingredients.

Calcium; Calcium is critical to take, but it can impede the absorption of zinc, iron, and manganese.

Zinc; Zinc can interfere with the uptake of amino acids and iron.

Magnesium; Magnesium can interfere with the uptake of calcium.

49. What Time of Day Should I Take My Supplements?

Most of your supplements can be taken with your largest meal of the day, which should contain some fat. Typically the largest meal is lunch or dinner; for me, it's lunch since I practice intermittent fasting. The most essential point is that they should be taken with food to help digestion and absorption.

However, some supplements are best taken without food or before bedtime to increase effectiveness. For example, SAM-e, a supplement used to treat mood disorders, should be taken on an empty stomach at minimum 30 minutes before consuming food. If taken with food, SAM-e's effectiveness is greatly diminished. Check the product label for how to take your dietary supplement.

50. What would a sample vitamin schedule look like?

Sample Vitamin Schedule

With breakfast
- B vitamins
- Multivitamin (properly dosed for age and sex) or prenatal multivitamin/folic acid
- Omega-3s
- Probiotics

With lunch
- Vitamin D (Don't take vitamin D at night because it pauses melatonin production and will interfere with sleep)
- Calcium

With dinner
- Vitamin C
- Iron

Before bed

♦ Fiber supplement (with a glass of water, research suggests it may improve sleep)

51. Can supplements be used to treat disease?

What do you do when a supplement knocks on your door? You in"vitamin"

According to the FDA, dietary supplements are intended to supplement the diet. They are not medicines intended to treat, diagnose, mitigate, prevent, or cure diseases. However, supplements can be used as part of a treatment plan for specific conditions under a healthcare professional's supervision.

52. What are probiotics and prebiotics?

Why did the bacteria cross the microscope? To get to the other slide.

Probiotics are bacteria found in foods such as yogurt and sauerkraut. Prebiotics are the fiber that probiotics feed on in foods such as whole grains, greens, onions, garlic, soybeans, artichokes, and bananas.

The human microbiome comprises bacteria, fungus, and other microorganisms that participate in food digestion, affect mental health, and nearly every other bodily process. Your microbiota can make up to 10% of your body weight (for example, I weigh 210 lbs. so I have around 21 pounds of bacteria in my body). We have approximately 300 to 500 bacterial species living within the human gastrointestinal system, comprising nearly 2 million genes (the microbiome). The majority of our microbiome lives here, as many as 400 trillion microbes.

The use of prebiotics and probiotics to treat medical disorders is called microbiome therapy. You don't need to take prebiotics for probiotics together, but taking them together will be more effective.

Adjusting your diet and taking probiotics and prebiotics can significantly positively impact your health. Most of the time, the helpful and unhelpful bacteria work together in your body and balance each other out. However, if you don't eat a balanced diet, the unhealthy bacteria can increase in population and cause dysbiosis, an imbalance in the gut microbial community associated with disease.

53. How do you know if you're taking the right supplements?

There are three ways to evaluate which supplements you should be taking. The first way to figure out what vitamins and supplements to take is to look carefully at the nutritional value of all the foods in your diet and see how close you are to the recommended daily uptake of the nutrients. The easiest way to do this is with your iPhone, which can process millions of times more information than the machines NASA used for the Moon landings.

A. Calorie Counter & Food Diary

Enter your nutritional and weight loss goals, plan your meals and monitor your adherence. Valuable features include scanning supermarket barcodes to get nutritional information while grocery shopping and tracking your macronutrients such as carbohydrates, protein, and fat. You can track your intake of 45 different nutrients. The user interface makes entering your food intake fast and easy, essential because people abandon a food diary app when it becomes too complicated.

B. Nutrients

It contains the nutritional info for a wide range of foods which makes tracking your food intake simple. One particular feature allows you to enter your recipes and get an instant dietary breakdown.

C. Shopwell

The Shopwell app helps you make healthy choices at the grocery store. Enter your fitness goals, nutritional requirements, and food sensitivities when setting up the app. Then, as you're shopping, scan the barcodes of items you're considering for information about the nutritional content, added sugar and sodium, and more.

D. Calorie Counter & Diet Tracker by MyFitnessPal

My Fitness Pal is one of the most straightforward, most intuitive, and popular apps for tracking your food intake for weight loss. It has a database of 5,000,000 foods and dishes you can use to log your meals quickly.

E. MyPlate Calories Tracker

It has a nutritional database of 2 million items. It includes tracking calories, macronutrients, and water intake and seeing if you're meeting your diet goals. You can generate graphs and charts that help you to visualize and assess your food habits.

The second way is to fill out medical questionnaires and provide them to your healthcare provider to do a clinical risk assessment and devise a supplement plan to meet your needs.

Sample Supplement Checklist

What happens when a computer doesn't get enough vitamin C?

It turns into a scurver!

Answer these questions and take this list to your healthcare professional to help them determine if you need blood tests for the final determination of supplements you may need. If you get blood and allergy tests, you can pair this list with your results to help you shop for supplements.

1. What medications are you currently taking?
(Medications may affect your recommended supplements.)
Medication name
2. What supplements are you currently taking?
3. Do you have food allergies?
4. Do you follow a specialized diet? For example, vegan, ovolactovegetarian, gluten-free, keto, paleo, etc.?
5. Do you have kidney or liver disease?
6. Do you care if the supplements are vegetarian or not?
7. Do you have any sensitivities to or try to avoid any of the following? (circle all that apply) Latex, Milk, Mushrooms, Bee Products, Gluten, Soy, Fish, Ragweed, Shellfish, Nightshades, Peanuts, Tree Nuts, _____
8. On average, how many servings of fresh fruit and vegetables do you eat in a day? (One serving of fresh fruit is equivalent to one apple or eight strawberries. One serving of vegetables is equal to a handful of broccoli.) 0 to 2, 3 to 5, 6 or more

9. How many servings of calcium-rich foods do you typically eat daily? (One serving of calcium-rich foods is equivalent to a fistful of spinach, one cup of milk, 3 to 4 cubes of cheese, or a handful of almonds.) 0 to 2, 3, 4, or more servings
10. Do you currently smoke or come into contact with second-hand smoke (tobacco or marijuana)? (Your vitamin requirements may vary if you smoke or are exposed to second-hand smoke.)
Yes or No.
11. On average, how many days a week do you drink alcoholic beverages? (Consuming high amounts of alcohol may impact your liver.) 0 to 1, 2 to 3, 4 or more
12. Have you had any genetic health testing? ((e.g., 23 and me™, Ancestry™, etc.) Bring a copy of your genetic health tests to your healthcare provider visit and this checklist.) Your test results can help your healthcare provider make recommendations specific to your needs.
Yes or No
13. Based on your genetic test, are you at increased risk of having lower levels of any nutrients?
None of these
Vitamin D
Omega 3
Vitamin C
Vitamin E
14. Are you at increased risk for any of these conditions based on your genetic test?
Osteoporosis or Osteopenia, Hypercholesterolemia, Macular Degeneration, Hemochromatosis, Cognitive Dysfunction, Thrombophilia
15. Do you participate in Intermittent Fasting?
Yes or No
16. Are you trying to lose more than 10 lbs.?
Yes or No
17. Do you track your daily steps? On average, how many steps are you taking per day?
I don't track my steps, Less than 5000, 5000-7500, 7500-10000, 10000, or more.
18. Do you regularly keep track of your daily steps?
(eg. Apple Health, Garmin, accelerometer, Fitbit, pedometer)

Yes or No

19. How many hours per week do you do vigorous or long-distance cardio (e.g., jogging, running, biking, swimming)? (Supplements can support movement and cardiovascular exercise to optimize your workout routine.)

Less than 2 hours, 2-3 hours, 3 to 4 hours, More than 4 hours

20. Which best describes your fitness or activity level? (If you exercise, supplements can support your joints and muscles.)

I never or rarely work out. I occasionally work out and/or would like to increase my workouts. I work out regularly. I am in great shape, and I work out all the time. I am an athlete or competitor.

21. Do you regularly engage in other exercises for more than 30 minutes at least three times a week?

I don't do any other exercise.
Yoga or Pilates
Power Walking
Strength or resistance training
Other

22. How sore are you after your workouts? (Supplements help you combat exercise-induced stress and improve recovery time.)

Maybe a little, but no complaints, Sometimes All of the time

23. Is your exposure to the sun limited daily? ((e.g., spending time indoors, use of sunscreen or protective clothing) Limited sun exposure and daily sunscreen usage can lead to Vitamin D) deficiency.

Yes or No

24. Do you have any of these skin conditions? (Some supplements help improve certain skin conditions.)

None
Eczema
Vitiligo
Psoriasis
Chronic cold sores

25. Are you experiencing BPH (an enlarged prostate)?

(BPH (Benign Prostatic Hyperplasia) is an enlargement of the prostate gland that can compress parts of the urinary tract.)
Yes or No
26. Do you experience any of the following?
None
Adrenal fatigue symptoms
Chronic aches and pains
27. Has anyone in your immediate family had any of these conditions? (Family history is an essential indicator of your future health)
None
Colon Cancer
Prostate Cancer
28. How are your mood and stress levels?
I have no complaints.
I'm stressed all of the time.
I would like to improve my mood
I am rarely happy, or I feel indifferent
I often feel tired and unable to focus
29. Do you often have any of these digestive problems? (Digestive disorders can have multiple causes.)
No complaints
Constipation
Bloating
Diarrhea
30. On average, how well do you sleep?
(Improving your quality of sleep is one way you can work to prevent developing chronic disease.)
I sleep well
When I try to sleep, my mind often races
I don't sleep well for another reason
My sleep is interrupted (snoring or waking up to urinate)
31. On average, how are your energy levels?
I usually have an energy slump. I'm always exhausted. I have no complaints.
32. Do you have any of these conditions related to your immune or cellular health?
None
Chronic Fatigue Syndrome

Lupus
Frequent colds or viral infections
Seasonal allergies
I have had or currently have cancer
Celiac Disease
33. Do you have any of these conditions related to your nervous system?
None
Vertigo
Age-related cognitive decline
Migraine Headaches
Fibromyalgia
34. Do you have any of these conditions related to your lung health?
None
Emphysema
Another lung condition
Asthma
Exercise-Induced Asthma
Chronic Obstructive Pulmonary Disease (COPD)
35. Do you have any of these conditions related to your eye, nose, and gum health?
None
Glaucoma
Cataracts
Sinusitis
Macular Degeneration
Gingivitis
36. Do you have any of these conditions related to your heart health?
None
High Triglycerides
Congestive Heart Failure
Atherosclerosis
High Cholesterol not taking statins
High Cholesterol and I am taking statins
High Blood Pressure
Angina
37. Do you have any of these conditions related to your joint and bone health?

None
Tendinitis
Rheumatoid Arthritis
Osteoarthritis
Osteoporosis
38. Are you interested in supporting your immune system during cold and flu season?
No or Yes
39. Do you have any conditions related to your stomach and digestive health?
None
Irritable Bowel Syndrome
Acid Reflux or Heartburn
Abdominal Pain
Indigestion
I've taken antibiotics in the past 12 months.
40. Do you have any blood sugar and endocrine health conditions?
None
Hyperthyroidism
High Blood Sugar or Type I/II Diabetes
Diabetic Retinopathy
Diabetic Neuropathy

The third and most accurate way is through blood lab tests which can detail your body's needs. Some tests your healthcare provider may use include;

    a. Vitamin panel blood test checks the levels of thirteen essential vitamins to identify any deficiencies and determine if supplements are needed.

    b. Heavy metals panel or heavy metal toxicity test can check for heavy metal poisoning with a blood test.

    c. Using blood or urine samples, oxidative stress can be measured indirectly by measuring the levels of DNA/RNA damage, lipid peroxidation, and protein oxidation/nitration in the sample.

    d. A blood test can check most of the hormone and neurotransmitter levels in your blood, such as thyroid, estrogen, testosterone, and cortisol levels.

e. A blood test can measure your immune system's response to particular foods by measuring the allergy-related antibody known as immunoglobulin E (IgE).

f. Signs of age-related cognitive decline can be assessed using the Short Test of Mental Status, the Montreal Cognitive Assessment (MoCA), or the Mini-Mental State Examination (MMSE).

g. Another option is home testing kits using stool and blood tests. These are cost-effective and sound options, including LetsGetChecked Micronutrient Test, Viome, and Rootine Blood Vitamin Test.

54. What is chelation?

A chelating agent is a substance that bonds with a mineral to create a more absorbable end product. Chelates are organic forms of essential trace minerals such as copper, iron, manganese, and zinc. Humans absorb, digest, and use mineral chelates better than inorganic minerals. Because it's difficult for your body to absorb some minerals such as zinc on its own efficiently, zinc is often attached to a chelating agent in supplements.

55. Where should I store my supplements?

Vitamins can lose their potency over time and should be stored at or below room temperature. If bottles sit on a shelf in a warm room or under direct sunlight, they may degrade even before expiration. Storage directions usually explained on the supplement label. In general, store your supplements in a cool, dry place with the lid sealed.

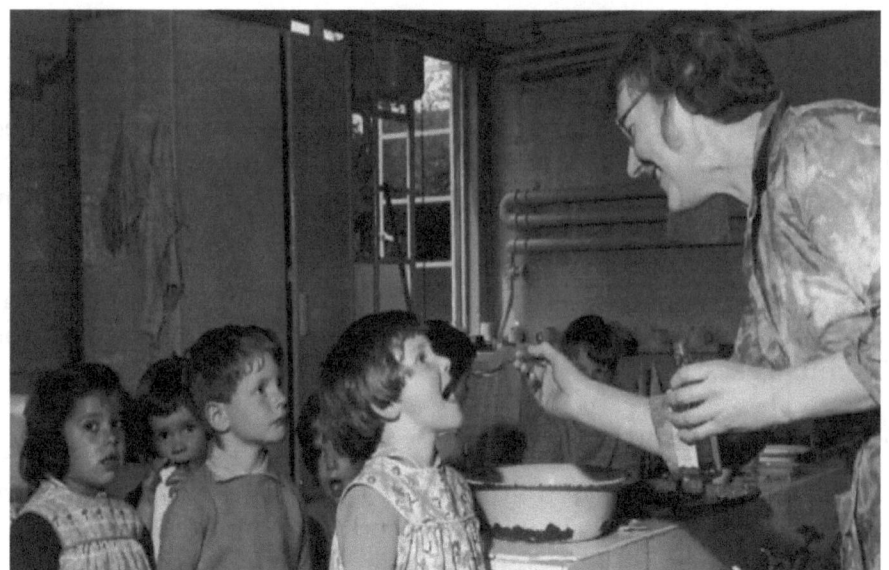
Children lining up to have their daily dose of Cod Liver Oil

56. How to get started with supplements?

Look for patterns in your day and consider how you can use existing habits to create new ones. The best way to start a new practice is to attach it to an existing one. For example, "I'll take my vitamins with my breakfast." but be specific; rather than saying you'll take your vitamins with breakfast, decide which supplements you'll take and when exactly, such as before you start eating. The more precise you are with your habits, the more likely you'll follow them.

Think of the story of Pavlov's dog. Pavlov fed his dogs every time he rang a bell. After being conditioned to the behavior, the dogs started salivating every time they heard the bell, even if the food was not present. We want to condition ourselves so that we don't have to think about taking supplements. Every morning before we eat, we automatically reach for our supplements and take them without thinking about it. Our morning routine is our most vital routine for many of us, so that's a great place to start on a new habit.

Use the 21/90 rule. Commit to a personal goal for 21 straight days. After three weeks of pursuing that goal, it should become a habit. Once you establish the routine, continue it for another ninety days. It should become a permanent lifestyle change if you can keep up something for three weeks and then ninety days.

The next step is to reduce the friction or difficulty of taking your supplements. The easier you make it for yourself, the more likely you'll stick to the habit. For example, rather than having your vitamins in their bottles in your medicine cabinet, you can get a pillbox and separate your vitamins for the whole month. It eliminates the need to locate each bottle individually, open and close each one, and figure out how many of each one to take.

You can also use your environment to prompt the behavior you're trying to form. Place your pillbox next to the glass of water you set out each night before sleeping. When you open your eyes in the morning and reach for your glass of water, your supplements will be in plain view providing a visual cue every morning.

Like they say in business school, KISS (keep it simple stupid). Start with the basics a multivitamin (properly dosed for age and sex) with iron, vitamin C, vitamin D, calcium, probiotics, omega fatty acids (Krill oil is ideal), and vitamin K2. Once you get started with these, you can add more to your regime as your finances allow. In taking your supplements, you'll notice some of them may have side effects (although rare), such as upset stomach. So you can start taking them exactly after you eat your breakfast rather than before, half before breakfast and a half after breakfast, or you can decide to take different forms of supplements such as gummies instead of pills. Once you get started with the basics, you can adjust your regime to your needs.

57. Which supplements should you keep, and which ones should you cut out if you need to save money?

I ran out of my Omega 3 supplement so I went to the store. The attendant was rude and threw the bottle at me as hard as he could. Fortunately, my injuries were super fish oil

Think of your supplements in three groups. The first group should include your essential supplements;

Multivitamin (for your sex and age group) with iron
Vitamin C
Vitamin D
Calcium
Probiotics,
Omega fatty acids (Krill oil is ideal)
Vitamin K2

The second group of supplements should support your personal and family health history. Creating a family and personal medical inventory will help you identify past, ongoing, and potential health problems to tailor a supplement plan specific to your medical needs. Your medical inventory should cover all major organ systems, including:

The urinary system: kidneys and bladder.
The cardiovascular system: heart and blood vessels
The skeletal system: bones and joints
The nervous system: brain and nerves
The respiratory system: lungs, sinuses, and bronchial passages
The digestive system: stomach, liver, and intestines
The immune system: thymus, spleen, and lymph nodes
The muscular system: muscles
The endocrine system: pancreas, glands, and hormones
Also, consider factors such as;
Eyes/ears/nose/throat
Diabetes/metabolism
Mental health/mood

The third group of supplements should address your current performance and fine-tune your health. These supplements are for optimizing your regimen. These supplements include anti-aging, weight loss, and improving brain function. These supplements are not required and tend to be more costly, so if you ever need to cut back, this is where you would want to cut back first.

Specifically, your supplement plan should address some of the most common chronic diseases to help slow their progression and improve their symptoms and outcome.

Examples include;
Bowel and Digestive Disorders
Brain Diseases like Alzheimer's and Parkinson's Disease

Cancers including Prostate, Breast, and Colon
Chronic Fatigue and Chronic Pain Syndromes
Diabetes and Metabolic Disorders
Lung Disorders like COPD and Asthma
Heart Diseases including Atherosclerosis and Heart Failure
Insomnia and Mood Disorders
Bone and Joint Disorders
Overweight and Obesity

58. What type of doctor should I see to have my blood tested?

Anita, an occupational therapist who was having joint pain, was referred to see a rheumatologist and was diagnosed with rheumatoid arthritis. He recommended she start taking magnesium as part of her treatment plan. So she started immediately, and within a week, she started cramping throughout her body. So she went to see her chiropractor see if it was a musculoskeletal problem. Her chiropractor did muscle testing (An applied kinesiology technique for diagnosing structural, muscular, chemical, and mental ailments.) on her and determined that her problem was caused by overdosing on magnesium. Her chiropractor adjusted her dosage of magnesium, and Anita's issues with the muscle cramping went away.

Regardless of the years of experience or training, no one can see what is in your blood without a blood test. Either doctor could have ordered blood tests and avoided any issues with the recommended supplements. Having a blood test completed may have also revealed other deficiencies that could be causing Anita's joint problems and possibly prevent future health issues related to vitamin deficiencies. Because typically, when someone is deficient in one nutrient, they're probably not eating a balanced diet and most likely lacking other nutrients.

Many types of doctors can order blood tests medical doctor (MD), naturopathic doctor (ND), doctor of osteopathy (DO), doctor of dental surgery (DDS), nurse practitioner (NP), chiropractor (DC), physician assistant (PA), and many more healthcare practitioners can refer out to and use a certified clinical lab (CLIA) to analyze blood for diagnostic purposes.

59. What supplements does Dr. Martinez most often recommend to patients?

I call it my "Kirkland Stack," which is the private label of the store Costco. Kirkland is a Scottish name meaning land belonging to the church and is the city name where Costco was headquartered. I like this brand because most of their supplements are USP certified, the gold standard for supplement quality. They're easily accessible as there are Costcos in many places (even some international locations under different names like Price Smart). They have the basics for anyone who wants to start taking supplements, and the price is second to none. For around $200, you can buy a year's supply of quality supplements that will cover most people's basic needs. One of the main barriers for people to get started with supplements is there are too many options, to the point where it makes people worry if they're making the right choice or missing something. Costco has simplified the supplement buying process with their team of experts stocking the basics, so you're unlikely to make the wrong choice when picking supplements.

Kirkland Stack
Daily multivitamin with iron (500 tablets) $20
Vitamin B complex super (500 tablets) $18.50
Vitamin C 1000mg (500 tablets) $20
Vitamin D 50mcg (600 softgels) $11.50
Vitamin E 180 mg (500 softgels) $15
Calcium citrate magnesium and zinc (500 tablets) $16
CoQ10 300 mg (100 softgels) $25
Krill oil 500 mg (160 softgels) $25
Probiotic (100 capsules) (10 strains with 10 billion viable cells is enough) $20
Total $170
+add (if you have joint issues) Glucosamine with MSM $20

The other company I like is Nature Made. Nature Made is affordable, USP certified, has a diverse product line, and is based in California. A good choice as you start fine-tuning your supplement regime and working towards high performance.

When taking supplements (day and night) or eating foods containing fat-soluble vitamins such as vitamins A, E, D, and K (foods like carrots, leafy green veggies, and legumes), pair them with a dietary fat such as olive oil, fish oil, coconut oil, or butter (In moderation). Dietary fats significantly increase the body's ability for nutrient absorption. An example would be having a salad with an olive oil-based dressing or taking your fish oil, krill oil, astaxanthin, or MCT coconut oil with your supplements.

60. What supplements does Dr. Martinez take?

The Mexican instructor at the gym knew a lot about protein supplements.

So one day, I approached him and said, "Jesus, show me the whey."

My daily Supplement Regime

Here is my Supplement list as an example (Unless specified, I take the recommended dose on each bottle.) My list is dynamic as yours should be and is constantly changing according to my health goals and needs. My list of supplements is built to counteract some of the common issues a 47-year-old ovolactovegetarian male may encounter, such as cognitive decline, erectile dysfunction, muscle mass loss, decreased testosterone, and general aging. Your list will reflect individual needs according to your age, lifestyle, eating habits, sex, and health goals.

I recently experienced a breakup with my girlfriend. Interestingly, one of the things she took during our dissolution was my supplements. She said she had never felt stronger or healthier, and her skin glowed. A properly regimented supplement stack can do wonders for your health and success. The healthier you are, the better able you'll be to compete in your daily life and excel in whatever activities you engage in.

For accelerated fat loss and muscle building, drink "Hardcore Juice" as your first meal, drink one additional 20-ounce serving if you are still hungry, and cut your eating window to four hours.

Hardcore Juice:

Use a Vitamix 64-ounce blender to blend the ingredients below and refrigerate in glass bottles.

1 teaspoon of MCT Oil (Fat burning Brain Booster)

1 tablespoon of Turmeric Powder (Anti-inflammatory, stabilizes blood sugar, good for heart, brain, and bones)

1/2 teaspoon of Ceylon Cinnamon (Anti-inflammatory, stabilizes blood sugar, good for heart, brain, and bones)

1 tablespoon of Cocoa Powder (Anti-inflammatory, stabilizes blood sugar, good for heart, brain, and bones)

1 teaspoon of pure Vanilla extract (Antioxidant, anticancer, anti-inflammatory, neuroprotective)

1 teaspoon Creatine Monohydrate Powder (Improve strength, increase lean muscle mass, and speed recovery after exercise)

1/2 teaspoon HMB Powder (Improve strength, increase lean muscle mass, and speed recovery after exercise, especially in older adults)

1/2 teaspoon Beta-Alanine (Increased exercise capacity, decreases muscle fatigue, antioxidant with immune-enhancing and anti-aging properties)

1 teaspoon Glutamine (Boosts immune system, rebuilds intestinal health, benefits leaky gut, spurs muscle growth and running speed, reduces sugar and carb cravings)

1 1/4 teaspoon L-Citrulline DL-Malate 2:1 (Increased nitric oxide production, enhanced endurance and exercise performance, reduced muscle soreness, support for cardiovascular health, ammonia clearance, and potential erectile function support)

1 teaspoon of Beet Powder (Improved athletic performance, reduced blood pressure, improved brain function, lowered risk of cancer, enhanced cardiovascular health, increased endurance and reduced fatigue, antioxidant properties, support for liver health, digestive health)

1 1/2 teaspoon Acacia Fiber (Lowers bad cholesterol levels, keeps blood sugar in check, prevents diabetes, and helps treat irritable bowel syndrome (IBS))

1 teaspoon of Bee Pollen (Anti-inflammatory, improved immunity, menopausal symptoms, and wound healing.)

1/2 teaspoon pf Royal Jelly (Anti-inflammatory, improved immunity, antioxidant properties, improved cognitive function, anti-tumor, blood sugar control, balances hormones, decreases cholesterol, and protects liver.)

4 tablespoons of collagen peptides (18 grams of protein) (Improve digestion, strengthen joints and bones, improve the health of hair, skin, nails, and cognitive function)

1 teaspoon Matcha Green Tea powder (Powerful antioxidant, increases cognitive function, cleans the liver, prevents cancer, weight loss, and improves cardiovascular health)

Optional add vegan protein powder, Greek yogurt, kefir, and/or high protein soy milk. If you're using vegan protein powder, add 20% more to account for decreased bioavailability. Use 1/2 gram of protein powder for every pound of body weight. For example, I weigh 200 lbs, so I consume 100 grams daily. I would add half of my daily protein requirement, 50 grams, to my Hardcore Juice.

Mix in 20 ounces of warm water (not from a plastic bottle) or warm soy milk for 30-60 seconds (mixing time is essential to promote the creation of EZ water).

Use your Hardcore Juice to take your morning supplements.

1. Calcium (1000-1200 mg as calcium carbonate) Most vegetarians are deficient in calcium. Calcium builds and maintains strong bones. The heart, muscles, and nerves also need calcium to function properly. 7/10 people are deficient.

2. Nicotinamide mononucleotide (NMN) (1g) NMN has been able to suppress age-associated weight gain, enhance energy metabolism and physical activity, improve insulin sensitivity, improve eye function, improve mitochondrial metabolism and prevent age-linked changes in gene expression.

3. Resveratrol (1g) Resveratrol has antioxidant and anti-inflammatory properties to protect you against diseases like cancer, diabetes, and Alzheimer's disease. The anti-inflammatory effects of resveratrol make it a good remedy for arthritis and skin inflammation.

4. Potato Starch (1 tablespoon) Helps to control hunger, improve digestion, and immune health, control blood sugar, and manage weight. (To be used if you're still feeling hungry when going out to eat or to a party.) Potato starch is also prebiotic, feeding beneficial gut bacteria. The fermentation of resistant starch in the colon produces short-chain fatty acids like butyrate, which is helpful for colon health and a healthy gut microbiome.

Brain boosting Supplements (generally one hour before starting work activities)

    1. Citicoline (500–2,000 mg) Improves cognition and prevents cognitive decline

    2. Theacrine (50 to 300 mg) Increases energy and improves cognitive function

    3. Pyrroloquinoline Quinone (PQQ) (20mg) Raises blood flow to the cerebral cortex, improving attention, thinking, and memory.

    4. L-Theanine (100-400 mg) Improves cognitive function, eases anxiety, stress, and reduces insomnia.

    5. Genius Mushrooms. A type of fungi that increases blood flow and oxygen levels to the brain, which improves memory and cognitive function.

Relaxation (taken in the morning to help promote a peaceful day)

    1. Bach Rescue Remedy (1 drop a day) Used to relieve anxiety, nervous tension, stress, agitation or despair and provide a sense of focus and calm.

MORNING Supplements (Taken with the first meal to increase absorption and boost performance for the day)

    1. Metformin (500 mg) (prescription) In 1918, scientists discovered that the medicinal herb French Lilac (Galega officinalis) contained guanidine, which could lower blood sugar. Medicines containing guanidine, such as Metformin, were developed to treat diabetes. In 1995, the FDA approved

Metformin for the treatment of diabetes. Since then, it has become the most widely prescribed medication for diabetes. Metformin is approved for the treatment of type 2 diabetes. However, it is also used off-label to treat polycystic ovarian syndrome (PCOS), infertility, weight reduction, diabetes prevention, pregnancy complications, and obesity. Recent Harvard studies suggest that Metformin may increase life expectancy by an average of ten years and slow aging by improving the body's responsiveness to insulin, antioxidant effects, and blood vessel health. Activated Protein Kinase (AMPK metabolic activator) (450 mg) is a non-prescription less effective alternative.

2. Multivitamin with Iron. Vegetarians often do not get 8-18mg of iron daily. A multivitamin covers many supplements (iron, b-vitamins, copper, zinc) so you can cut down on the number of pills you take and replace the need to take a b-complex if you decide to cut back.

3. Vitamin A (3000-10,000 IU as retinyl palmitate) If you aren't consuming organ meats such as beef kidney, liver, or heart, then you're not going to get sufficient amounts of vitamin A in your diet. You can't get vitamin A from plants, and vegetables such as carrots won't help because they have beta-carotene instead of vitamin A. Vegetarians should take vitamin A because beta-carotene is poorly converted into vitamin A. Half of the population is deficient in this vitamin.

Don't take vitamin A supplements without consulting with a doctor if you have kidney disease, liver disease, or drink heavily.

4. Vitamin B-complex. Vitamin B-complex is a must for people like myself who eat a vegan and vegetarian plant-based diet which is typically deficient in B-vitamins. Vitamin B-complex relieves stress, boosts cognitive performance, and reduces symptoms of depression and anxiety.

5. Vitamin C (500-1000 mg as Ascorbic acid or liposomal) Vitamin C is the safest supplement you can take. It is used for collagen and connective tissue formation, making glutathione, the most potent antioxidant in the body, and preventing free radical damage. Vitamin C is heat-sensitive, so heating vegetables and fruits will destroy it. Take higher doses of vitamin C when you're sick. Half of the population is deficient.

6. Vitamin D (1,000 mg per 25 lbs of body weight) Vitamin D helps regulate the amount of calcium and phosphate in the body needed to keep bones, teeth and muscles healthy. Because most of us work indoors, most people are deficient. Up to 9/10 people are deficient in this vitamin.

7. Vitamin E (400 IU as D-Alpha-Tocopherol) Naturally sourced vitamin E is called d-alpha-tocopherol and is the preferred form of vitamin E transported and used by the liver. The synthetically produced form is labeled as dl-alpha-tocopherol and made from petroleum products. The RDA for vitamin E is 15 mg, but the upper tolerable intake level (UL) for vitamin E is 1,000 mg (1,500 IU). Research shows the optimal dose for disease prevention and treatment for adults is 400 to 800 IU per day. 8/10 people are deficient.

8. Vitamin K2 (100 mcg) It's difficult to get enough of this vitamin in your daily diet. Vitamin K2 activates a protein that helps calcium bind to bones, improving bone density and reducing the risk of bone fractures.

9. Probiotic (10 to 20 billion colony-forming units (CFU) Probiotics provide a wide variety of benefits against a range of health conditions, including allergies, arthritis, asthma, cancer, mental issues, and digestive problems. I take it to help keep my microbiome healthy.

10. Astaxanthin (10mg) Protects cells from damage, improves immune functions, athletic performance, aging skin, and reduces muscle soreness from exercise. It also helps with the absorption of fat-soluble vitamins.

11. Pycnogenol (pine bark, 400mg) Improves circulation, lowers blood pressure, and has anti-aging benefits.

12. Coenzyme Q10 (CoQ10) (300mg) It improves heart health, regulates blood sugar, assists in preventing and treating cancer, reduces the frequency of migraines, and reduces the oxidative damage that leads to muscle fatigue, skin damage, and brain and lung diseases.

13. Chlorella (5 grams) A good source of several vitamins, minerals, and antioxidants, it detoxifies the body and improves cholesterol and blood sugar levels.

14. Odorless Garlic Extract (1200mg) Lowers blood pressure, improves circulation, is an antioxidant, and contains neuroprotection properties.

15. Epigallocatechin Gallate (EGCG) (400 mg) Green tea extract, reduces inflammation, promotes weight loss, and helps prevent heart and brain disease.

16. Silicea (9-14 mg) Promotes collagen production, the body's most abundant protein, helps rebuild bones, skin, and joints.

17. Sea Kelp (500 mcg Iodine supplement) High in minerals and antioxidants, boosts energy, and improves muscle recovery.

18. Ashwagandha (1000 mg) is an adaptogenic herb clinically shown to help reduce stress, regulate cortisol levels, enhance focus, memory, and mental stamina, and reduce irritability and stress-related cravings. Improves sleep, lowers blood glucose levels and triglycerides, improves sexual function in women, supports heart health increases VO2 max levels, which is the maximum amount of oxygen you take in during physical exertion. Recent studies show that ashwagandha can increase testosterone levels in men by 10-15%, increasing strength and muscle size in men and not female participants.

NIGHT (Take with your last meal)

1. Metformin (2nd dose a day as needed) (500 mg) (prescription) Reduces fat storage, increases insulin sensitivity (to lower blood glucose), reduces cholesterol/triglyceride production, suppresses chronic inflammation, anti-aging, and increases lifespan.

2. Dehydroepiandrosterone (DHEA) (100mg) Improves cognitive function, erectile function, and helps prevent obesity.

3. L-Arginine (1-2 grams) & L-Ornithine (500-1000mg) (1 pill best taken together) Lowers blood pressure (if you take a blood pressure medication talk to your doctor before using it,) and treats erectile dysfunction. L-ornithine reduces fatigue and improves measures of athletic performance such as speed, strength, and power. Taking L-ornithine in combination with L-arginine also enhances strength and power in weightlifters.

4. Alpha-Lipoic Acid (225mg) & Acetyl L-Carnitine (525mg) (Combined in 1 pill) Alpha-lipoic acid is a potent antioxidant that reduces inflammation and skin aging, improves nerve function, lowers heart disease risk factors, and slows memory loss disorders.) Acetyl l-carnitine boosts your brain, mood, endurance, memory, strength and helps your body burn fat and recover from a workout.

5. Gamma-Aminobutyric Acid (GABA) (750mg) Improves mood, relieves anxiety, and improves sleep.

6. Glutamine (1000mg) Speeds muscle recovery and promotes muscle growth.

7. Magnesium Glycinate (400 mg) Essential for maintaining good health and plays a crucial role in everything from exercise performance to heart health and brain function. 50% of people are deficient.

8. Glutathione (1000mg) Promotes tissue building and repair, and immune system function.

9. Hyaluronic Acid (100 mg) Alleviates dry skin, reduces the appearance of fine lines and wrinkles and speeds up wound healing.

10. Krill Oil (500 mg) An excellent alternative to fish oil which often has contaminants and spoils quickly. Krill oil is high in omega-3 fatty acids that improve heart health, fight inflammation, and support brain and nervous system health.

11. Melatonin as needed (5mg) According to the National Institute of Health {NIH), Melatonin is the primary hormone regulating our sleep-wake cycle, the circadian rhythm. It is found in high concentrations in the mitochondria and is a mitochondria-targeted antioxidant, which indicates that it is an anti-aging mechanism. Melatonin is the most effective lipophilic antioxidant, proven twice as effective as vitamin E at preventing oxidative stress and cellular apoptosis.

I have been using the above supplements for many years, making adjustments as my health needs changed with good results. I had my stool tested for deficiencies, and switched from the above to a custom supplement program based on the results. I tried this regime for three months, and I had no noticeable improvements. I did, however, lose muscle mass and size as I was not taking as many muscle-building supplements. The cost of the custom program was $150 a month, and the cost of my usual supplement program was around $400 a month. There was a substantial savings and, as mentioned, no noticeable difference. I decided to go back to my self-designed supplement stack because it covered more areas than the custom program.

(Custom program provided to me by Viome after stool sample)
Turkey Tail Fruit Body Extract 71 mg / day
Nicotinamide Riboside (NR) 199 mg / day
N-Acetyl-L-Cysteine(NAC) 293 mg / day
Lycopene 79 mg / day
L. salivarius Ls-33 500 million CFU / day
Gamma Oryzanol 32 mg / day
Coenzyme Q-10 (CoQ10) 81 mg / day
Bacillus subtilis DE111 1 billion CFU / day
Pantethine 399 mg / day
L. plantarum Lp-115 1 billion CFU / day
Betaine Hydrochloride 403 mg / day

Beet Root Juice 600 mg / day
Boswellia Serrata Gum Extract 120 mg / day
Bacillus coagulans SANK 70258 500 million CFU / day
B. longum sp infantis Bi-26 500 million CFU / day
Lactococcus lactis LI-23 500 million CFU / day
Mastic Gum Extract 148 mg / day
Inositol 148 mg / day
L. acidophilus NCFM 500 million CFU / day
Pyrroloquinoline Quinone (PQQ) 9 mg / day
Zinc Carnosine 52 mg / day
Butyrate 763 mg / day
Creatine 279 mg / day
Pygeum Bark Extract 57 mg / day
Psyllium Husk Fiber 1600 mg / day
Saw Palmetto Berry Extract 192 mg / day
L. plantarum 299v 2.5 billion CFU / day
Fisetin 60 mg / day Apple Pectin 1600 mg / day
Inulin 500 mg / day
Fructo-oligosaccharides(FOS) 1700 mg / day
B. breve Bb-03 1 billion CFU / day
Tribulus Terrestris Extract 205 mg / day
Pumpkin Seed 330 mg / day
L. rhamnosus GG (ATCC 53103) 2.5 billion FU / day
B. animalis ssp lactis HN019 1 billion CFU / day
L-Glutamine 721 mg / day
Acetyl L-Carnitine 403 mg / day

Although this extensive list may cause you to think that supplements are one of the most critical parts of ideal health, they still represent a small overall component of your health plan. This diagram reminds us of where we need to invest our resources to achieve optimal health.

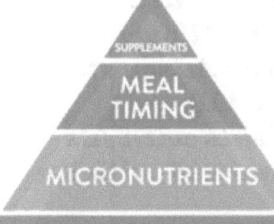

61. How much is too much?

The RDA gives you the minimum values of nutrients to avoid disability, but most of us could use more than the RDA, depending on our needs. When taking supplements, more is not always better. In particular, be careful with fat-soluble vitamins A, D, E, and K, as they can build up in your body and become toxic and even lethal.

Vitamin or Mineral	Recommended Dietary Allowance (RDA) or Adequate Intake (AI) Nutrients with AIs are marked with an (*)	Upper Tolerable Limit (UL) The highest amount you can take without risk
Boron	Not determined.	20 mg/day
Calcium	Age 19-50: 1,000 mg/day Women age 51+: 1,200 mg/day Men age 71+: 1,200 mg/day	Age 19-50: 2,500 mg/day Age 51 and up: 2,000 mg/day
Chloride	Age 19-50: 2,300 mg/day Age 50-70: 2,000 mg/day Age 70 and older: 1,800 mg/day	3,600 mg/day
Choline (Vitamin B complex)	Women: 425 mg/day * Men: 550 mg/day *	3,500 mg/day
Copper	900 micrograms/day	10,000 mcg/day
Fluoride	Men: 4 mg/day * Women: 3 mg/day*	10 mg/day

Folic Acid (Folate)	400 mcg/day	1,000 mcg/day *This applies only to synthetic folic acid in supplements or fortified foods. There is no upper limit for folic acid from natural sources.*
Iodine	150 mcg/day	1,100 mcg/day
Iron	*Men:* 8 mg/day *Women age 19-50:* 18 mg/day *Women age 51 and up:* 8 mg/day	45 mg/day
Magnesium	*Men age 19-30:* 400 mg/day *Men age 31 and up:* 420 mg/day *Women age 19-30:* 310 mg/day *Women age 31 and up:* 320 mg/day	350 mg/day *This applies only to magnesium in supplements or fortified foods. There is no upper limit for magnesium in food and water.*
Manganese	*Men:* 2.3 mg/day * *Women:* 1.8 mg/day*	11 mg/day
Molybdenum	45 mcg/day	2,000 mcg/day
Nickel	*Not determined*	1 mg/day

Phosphorus	700 mg/day	*Up to age 70:* 4,000 mg/day *Over age 70:* 3,000 mg/day
Selenium	55 mcg/day	400 mcg/day
Sodium	*Age 19-50:* 1,500 mg/day * *Age 51-70:* 1,300 mg/day * *Age 71 and up:* 1,200 mg/day *	2,300 mg/day
Vanadium	*Not determined*	1.8 mg/day
Vitamin A	*Men:* 900 mcg/day *Women:* 700 mcg/day	3,000 mcg/day
Vitamin B3 (Niacin)	*Men:* 16 mg/day *Women:* 14 mg/day	35 mg/day *This applies only to niacin in supplements or fortified foods. There is no upper limit for niacin in natural sources.*

Vitamin B6	*Men age 19-50:* 1.3 mg/day *Men age 51 up:* 1.7 mg/day *Women age 19-50:* 1.3 mg/day *Women age 51 up:* 1.5 mg/day	100 mg/day
Vitamin C	*Men:* 90 mg/day *Women:* 75 mg/day	2,000 mg/day
Vitamin D (Calciferol)	*Age 1-70:* 15 mcg/day (600 IU or international unit) * *Age 70 and older:* 20 mcg/day (800 IU) *	100 mcg/day (4,000 IU)
Vitamin E (alpha-tocopherol)	22.4 IU/day (15 mg/day)	1,500 IU/day (1,000 mg/day) *This applies only to vitamin E in supplements or fortified foods. There is no upper limit for vitamin E from natural sources.*
Zinc	*Men:* 11 mg/day *Women:* 8 mg/day	40 mg/day

62. What are the best Supplements for each category?

What do you call a Mexican bodybuilder who has run out of supplements?
No Whey Jose

Supplements for Exercise and Athletic Performance
Antioxidants (vitamin C, vitamin E, and coenzyme Q10)
Arginine
Beetroot or beet juice
Beta-alanine
Beta-hydroxy-beta-methylbutyrate (HMB)
Betaine
Branched-chain amino acids (BCAAs)
Caffeine
Citrulline
Creatine
Deer antler velvet
Dehydroepiandrosterone (DHEA)
Ginseng
Glutamine
Iron
Protein
Quercetin
Ribose
Sodium bicarbonate
Tart or sour cherry
Tribulus terrestris

Muscle mass and strength
Creatine
Protein powders
Amino acids
BCAA
Androstenedione
DHEA
HMB
Tribulus terrestris
Vanadium

Boron
Zinc

Endurance and energy
Ma huang
B-complex
Bee pollen
Blue green algae
Siberian ginseng (ciwujia)
Cordyceps sinensis
Ginseng
Royal jelly
OKG (ornithine alpha-ketoglutarate)
Gamma-oryzanol aka rice bran oil
MCT oil

Recovery
Glucosamine & Chondroitin
Sports drinks
Glycerol
B-complex
Glutamine
Zinc
Beta-sitosterol

Weight-Loss Dietary Supplements
African mango (Irvingia gabonensis)
Beta-glucans
Bitter orange (Citrus aurantium L.)
Caffeine (as added caffeine or from guarana, kola nut, yerba maté, or other herbs)
Calcium
Carnitine
Chitosan
Chromium
Coleus forskohlii
Conjugated linoleic acid
Fucoxanthin
Garcinia cambogia (hydroxycitric acid)
Glucomannan
Green coffee bean extract (Coffea arabica, Coffea canephora, Coffea robusta)

Green tea (Camellia sinensis) and green tea extract
Guar gum
Hoodia (Hoodia gordonii)
Probiotics
Pyruvate
Raspberry ketone
Vitamin D
White kidney bean (Phaseolus vulgaris)
Yohimbe (Pausinystalia yohimbe)

Alzheimer's Disease
Fish Oil/Omega-3s
Ginkgo Biloba
B-vitamins
Curcumin
Melatonin

Covid-19
Andrographis
Echinacea
Elderberry (European Elder)
Ginseng
Magnesium
Melatonin
N-acetylcysteine
Omega-3 fatty acids
Probiotics
Quercetin
Selenium
Vitamin C
Vitamin D
Vitamin E
Zinc

Brain Health
Ashwaghanda
Bacopa Monnieri
Gingko Biloba
Ginseng
Huperzine A
Nootropics
Omega-3 Fatty Acids

Phenibut
Rhodiola Rosea
Vinpocetine

Diabetes
Alpha-Lipoic Acid
Chromium
Cinnamon
Bitter Melon
Various Chinese Herbal Medicines
Fenugreek
Ginseng
Milk Thistle
Sweet Potato
Magnesium
Omega-3s
Selenium
Vitamin C
Vitamin D

Eye Conditions
Omega-3 Fatty Acids
Zinc
Beta-Carotene
Lutein and Zeaxanthin
Vitamins C and E

Menopause
Phytoestrogens
Black Cohosh
DHEA
Dong Quai
Vitamin E
Evening Primrose Oil
Ginseng
Kava
Melatonin
Wild yam

Osteoarthritis
Glucosamine and Chondroitin Sulfate
DMSO and MSM

SAMe
Boswellia Serrata
Arnica topical gel
Comfrey Extract gel
Capsicum Extract gel
Hyaluronic Acid

Primary Mitochondrial Disorders
Alpha-lipoic acid (ALA)
Arginine
Carnitine
Citrulline
Coenzyme Q10
Creatine
Folinic Acid
Niacin
Riboflavin
Thiamin
Vitamin C
Vitamin E
Vitamin K

Rheumatoid Arthritis
Omega-3 Fatty Acids
Gamma-Linolenic Acid (GLA)
Probiotics
Thunder God Vine
Cat's Claw
Deer or Elk Antler Velvet
Feverfew
Flaxseed Oil
Green-Lipped Mussel
Rose Hip
Willow Bark Extract

Anti-Aging
Curcumin
Epigallocatechin gallate (EGCG)
Collagen
Coenzyme Q10 (CoQ10)
Nicotinamide riboside (NR) and nicotinamide mononucleotide (NMN)

Crocin
Vitamin C
Vitamin E
Theanine
Rhodiola
Astragalus
Fisetin
Resveratrol
Sulforaphane

Supplements for Heart Health
Coenzyme Q10 (Co Q10)
Psyllium fiber
Omega-3 fatty acids
Magnesium
L-Carnitine
Green tea
Garlic
Inositol
Folate
Grape seed extract
Vitamin D
Red yeast rice

Supplements for Immune System Support
Vitamin D
Zinc
Vitamin C
Elderberry
Medicinal mushrooms
Astragalus
Selenium
Garlic
Andrographis
Licorice
Pelargonium sidoides
B complex vitamins
Curcumin
Echinacea
Propolis
Vitamin E

Supplements for Bone Health
Vitamin K2
Calcium
Vitamin D
Magnesium
Isoflavones
Vitamin C
Vitamin D
Bone meal (calcium, phosphorous, minerals)
Collagen peptides
Nitric Oxide
Omega-3 fatty acids
Sulfur (from Methylsulfonylmethane, sulfur amino acids, and green leafy veggies)
Glycosaminoglycans (chondroitin and hyaluronic acid)
Phytonutrients (Boswellia serrata, EGCG, lignans, genistein, phytoestrogens, turmeric etc.)

Supplements for Skin Care
Omega-3 fatty acids
Fern Extract
GLA Oils
Zinc
Calcium
Vitamins (A, C, and E)
Phytonutrients
CoQ10
Biotin
Hyaluronic Acid
Curcumin
Selenium

Supplements for Gastrointestinal Health
Probiotics
Prebiotics
Licorice
peppermint oil
Chamomile
Ginger
L-glutamine
Psyllium

Artichoke leaf extract
Inulin
Collagen
Wormwood
Moringa Leaf Powder
Marshmallow Root
Bentonite Clay

Supplements for Male Health
Vitamin D
Magnesium
Boron
Omega-3's
Saw Palmetto Extract
vitamin E.
L-arginine.
Pycnogenol.
Yohimbe /yohimbine.
Tribulus terrestris.
Eurycoma longifolia (tongkat ali)
Vitamin C
Niacin (vitamin B3)
Folic acid (vitamin B9)
Horny goat weed
Yohimbe
Red ginseng
DHEA
Citrulline
Arginine

Supplements for Support during Cancer
Omega-3 fatty acids (from Flax seed)
Garlic
Ginger
Green tea
Selenium
Turmeric
Vitamin B complex
Vitamin E
Resveratrol

More than 100 types of mushrooms are used to treat cancer.
Some of the more common ones are Ganoderma lucidum (reishi),
Trametes versicolor or Coriolus versicolor (turkey tail),
Lentinus edodes (shiitake), and
Grifola frondosa (maitake)

63. What are the top 5 Supplement Websites?

1. National Institute of Health Office of Dietary Supplements (www.ods.od.nih.gov)
2. WebMD has a tool to help you assess which supplements are best for you (www.webmd.com)
3. ConsumerLab.com (www.consumerlab.com)
4. Council for Responsible Nutrition (www.crnusa.org)
5. Nutrition Action Network

64. What are the top Supplement Brands?

Best overall vitamin brand: Nature Made
Best range of vitamin types: MegaFood
Best vitamin subscription brand: Ritual
Best personalized vitamin brand: Persona
Best personalized vitamin subscription brand: Care/of
Best vegan vitamin brand: Garden of Life
Best vitamin brand for athletes: Klean Athlete
Best bulk vitamin brand: Kirkland Signature
Best vitamin brand for purity: Thorne Research
Best budget vitamin brand: Amazon Elements
Best vitamin brand for gluten-free options: Standard Process
Best vitamin brand for omega supplements: Nordic Naturals
Best vitamin brand for range of supplements: Life Extension
Best vitamin brand for gummies: SmartyPants

Best brands according to ConsumerLab.com
Top-rated Supplement Brands on Overall Consumer Satisfaction
By Sales Channel:

Catalog/Internet Brand: Life Extension
Discount/Warehouse Brand: Kirkland (Costco)
Food/Drug/Mass -- Broad Product Line: Nature Made
Food/Drug/Mass -- Narrow Product Line: HPF Cholestene
Grocery Store Brand: Trader Darwin (Trader Joe's)
Healthcare Practitioner Brand: Designs for Health
Health Food Store Brand: Yerba Prima
Pharmacy Brand: CVS
Vitamin Store Brand: Vitamin Shoppe
Canadian Brand: Webber Naturals

By Type of Supplement:
Calcium: Citracal
CoQ10: Life Extension
Joint Health: Kirkland (Costco)
Magnesium: Life Extension
Melatonin: Natrol
Multivitamin: Life Extension
Omega-3s: Carlson
Probiotic: Garden of Life
Vitamin C: Ester-C
Vitamin D: Kirkland (Costco)

By Supplement Focus:
Apple Cider Vinegar: Bragg
Astaxanthin: BioAstin
Collagen: Great Lakes Gelatin Co.
Mushrooms: Real Mushrooms
Red Yeast Rice: HPF Cholestene
Sports Nutrition: Optimum Nutrition
Vitamin C: Ester-C

Top-rated Supplement Merchants on Overall Consumer Satisfaction

By Sales Channel:
Catalog/Internet: Life Extension
Grocery Store: Trader Joe's
Mass Market: Target
Online Multi-Category Retailer: Amazon.com
Online Supplement Retailer: Vitacost
Pharmacy: Local Pharmacies

Practitioner Line Merchant: Healthcare Practitioners' Offices
Vitamin Store: The Vitamin Shoppe
Warehouse Store: Costco

Best personalized vitamins
Best overall: Hum Nutrition
Most informative: Care/of
Widest selection: Persona Nutrition
Best budget option: Nurish
Best for accuracy: Viome
Best for athletes: Gainful

65. Do I need to take protein powder as part of my supplement program?

What did the gym goer say to their trainer when asked if they'd consider switching to a protein powder supplement? No whey!

No, most Americans are not deficient in protein. You can easily get the protein you need from natural sources, such as eggs, animal meats, beans, dairy, nuts, seeds, and whole grains. Most people are deficient in vitamins and minerals and benefit from other supplements. However, athletes and people on modified diets benefit from protein powder because they typically need more protein, plus it's convenient. For example, Aharon, a vegetarian college football player, needs to build muscle. To increase muscle mass in combination with physical activity, a person should eat 0.5 to 0.8 grams of protein per pound of body weight. Adding protein powder was an easy way to add more protein to his diet without cutting out vegetables from his diet to make room for the protein.

If you're going to add protein powder, consider using vegan protein powders, as they have fewer toxins than animal-based protein powders. Researchers have found that many protein powders contained:

- Heavy metals (lead, arsenic, cadmium, and mercury).
- Bisphenol-A (BPA, used to make plastic).
- Pesticides.
- Other contaminants linked to cancer and other health conditions.

People from various regions look, eat, behave, and cook in a manner that directly affects their health. The environment, media, culture, lifestyle, and economic status affect people's access to proper nutrition. Every part of the world has a specific set of challenges that causes specific vitamin deficiencies and benefits that causes a lack thereof. Understanding those unique needs will help better support a person's individual nutrient needs. To get the nutrients we need each day, we would need to consume over twenty pounds of food per day. For most people, this is impossible.

Along with over-farming that causes soil nutrient deficiencies, most experts believe that most people benefit from some supplementation as the quality of nutrition changes and we live accelerated lifestyles. Nutrient supplementation will become the standard, and people will seek to maximize their supplement regime by testing bodily fluids. To reach optimal physical and intellectual performance, we must give our body what it needs. Slight differences will determine who we are, how healthy we are, and how successful we ultimately are.

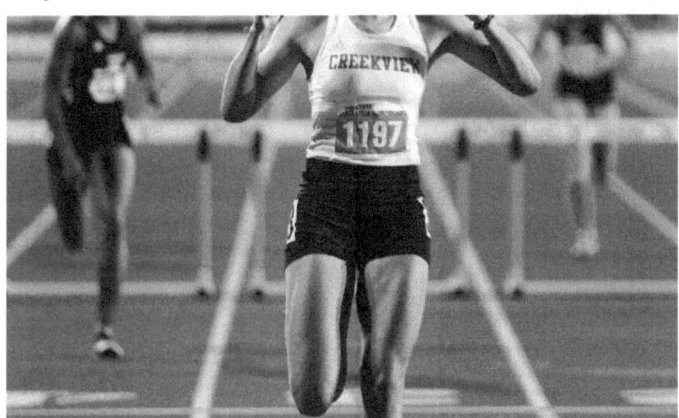

66. Most commonly used supplements.

Courtesy of the U.S. National Institue of Health (NIH)
5-HTP (5-hydroxytryptophan)

5-Hydroxytryptophan, also known as oxitriptan, is a naturally occurring amino acid and chemical precursor as well as a metabolic intermediate in the biosynthesis of the neurotransmitter serotonin.

Does it work?

Research suggests that 5-HTP can improve symptoms of fibromyalgia, including pain, anxiety, morning stiffness, and fatigue. Many people with fibromyalgia have low levels of serotonin, and doctors often prescribe antidepressants. Like antidepressants, 5-HTP raises levels of serotonin in the brain.

Is it safe?

When taken by mouth: It is possibly safe to take 5-HTP in doses of up to 400 mg daily for up to one year. The most common side effects include heartburn, stomach pain, nausea, vomiting, diarrhea, drowsiness, sexual problems, and muscle problems. Large doses of 5-HTP, such as 6-10 grams daily, are possibly unsafe.

A

Acai

They're Nutrient-Dense. Acai berries have a unique nutritional profile for a fruit, as they're somewhat high in fat and low in sugar.

Does it work?

So how exactly does acai berry work for weight loss? Acai berries have appetite suppression qualities; they are rich in fiber and also have a positive impact on the digestive system. Thus they help the body to process foods better and burn fat more efficiently in turn making it easier to lose weight.

Is it safe?

Acai pulp appears to be safe when consumed in the amounts commonly used in foods; however, drinking unprocessed acai juice has been linked to an illness called American trypanosomiasis (also known as Chagas disease). Consuming acai might affect MRI test results.

Artichoke Leaf Extract

The globe artichoke (Cynara cardunculus var. scolymus), also known by the names French artichoke and green artichoke in the U.S., is a variety of a species of thistle cultivated as a food.

Does it work?
Artichoke leaf extract may have a positive effect on cholesterol levels. A large review in over 700 people found that supplementing with artichoke leaf extract daily for 5–13 weeks led to a reduction in total and "bad" LDL cholesterol.

Is it safe?
Consuming artichoke extract is generally considered safe, with few side effects reported. However, there is limited data available. Risks include: Potential allergies: Some people may be allergic to artichokes and/or artichoke extract.

Arnica Topical Gel
Arnica is an herb sometimes used to flavor foods. It can be poisonous when consumed in larger amounts. Arnica gel can be applied to the skin for osteoarthritis. The active chemicals in arnica may reduce swelling, decrease pain, and act as antibiotics.

Does it work?
Possibly Effective for Osteoarthritis. Applying an arnica gel (A. Vogel Arnica Gel, Bioforce AG) twice daily for 3 weeks can reduce pain and stiffness and improve function in people with osteoarthritis in the hand or knee. It might work as well as ibuprofen.

Is it safe?
Arnica is generally safe when used on the skin. However, using it for a long time may irritate the skin, causing eczema, peeling, blisters, or other skin conditions. Arnica should not be used on broken skin, such as leg ulcers.

Activated Charcoal
Activated charcoal is used to treat poisonings, reduce intestinal gas (flatulence), lower cholesterol levels, prevent hangover, and treat bile flow problems (cholestasis) during pregnancy.

Does it work?
While activated charcoal is safe to consume in some cases, there is no evidence that it promotes weight loss, and nutrition experts do not recommend it for this purpose. In addition, it may cause side effects.

Is it safe?
When used to treat a poisoning or overdose, activated charcoal is usually safe, but it needs to be administered only in a healthcare facility. Side effects are more likely when it is used on a long-term basis to treat conditions like excess gas.

African Mango (see Weight Loss)
African mango seed extract is claimed to curb the formation of fat tissue.

Does it work?
African mango might help you lose a very small amount of weight.

Is it safe?
African mango seems to be safe, but its safety hasn't been well studied. It can cause headache, sleeping problems, flatulence, and gas.

Alfalfa
Alfalfa is a fiber-rich food and may help to control blood sugar levels by slowing the absorption of glucose into the intestines. As a result, it may help to control diabetes and prediabetes. Plant compounds called saponins lower the absorption of cholesterol in the intestines.

Does it work?
According to the USDA Nutrient Database, one cup of alfalfa sprouts has only 8 calories but delivers 0.2 grams fat, 0.7 grams carbohydrate, 0.6 grams fiber, and 1.3 grams protein. Alfalfa's rich soluble fiber content may help reduce cholesterol and aid in weight loss by increasing satiety.

Is it safe?
When taken by mouth: Alfalfa leaves are possibly safe when used short-term. But taking alfalfa in high doses or long-term is likely unsafe. Long-term use might cause reactions similar to the autoimmune disease called lupus in some people.

Aloe Vera
Aloe vera, or Aloe barbadensis, is a thick, short-stemmed plant that stores water in its leaves. It is best known for treating skin injuries, but it also has several other uses that could potentially benefit health.

Does it work?
Taking a spoonful of aloe vera before a meal helps the digestive system and promotes weight loss. It helps boost metabolism which in turn enables the body to burn fat. Presence of Vitamin B in aloe vera helps convert fat present in the body into energy and therefore aids weight loss.

Is it safe?
Is aloe vera safe? It's safe for most people to use aloe vera topically for minor skin care concerns. Generally, it's well tolerated, though skin irritations and allergic reactions are possible. Never use aloe vera or any severe cuts or burns.

Anabolic Steroids
Anabolic steroids, also known more properly as anabolic androgenic steroids, are steroidal androgens that include natural androgens like testosterone as well as synthetic androgens that are structurally related and have similar effects to testosterone.

Does it work?
Anabolic steroids can remain in the body anywhere from a couple of days to about a year. Steroids have become popular because they may improve endurance, strength, and muscle mass. However, research has not shown that steroids improve skill, agility, or athletic performance.

Is it safe?
There is no 'safe' dose of an anabolic steroid. If you continue to use steroids, despite health warnings and your doctors advice, however, keep the dose to an absolute minimum and take breaks from using the steroids.

Andrographis (see COVID-19)
Based on in silico investigations, the chemical constituents from turmeric like cyclocurcumin and curcumin and from Andrographis paniculata like andrographolide and dihydroxy dimethoxy flavone, significantly binding with the active site of SARS CoV-2 main protease, may produce significant activity and be useful for further development.

Does it work?

Andrographis paniculata (AP) is an herb used traditionally in Indian and Chinese medicine for several conditions, including the common cold. COVID is a disease that can cause symptoms like the common cold including sinus congestion, sore throat, fever, and cough. There is no research yet on treating COVID with AP. Some studies in cells found that AP may have anti-inflammatory effects and help the immune system, the body's way of fighting off infections.

Is it safe?
The amount of AP used for the common cold in research studies ranged from 450 mg to almost 2,000 mg of AP extract daily (divided into 3 to 4 doses) for 5 to 7 days. Side effects were rare and mild. 2-6 Doses of up to 6 grams daily for 7 days have been used with apparent safety.6 In the one prevention study, 200 mg per day (in divided doses) was used for 3 months, but more long-term studies are needed to know what the best dose of AP is for prevention.

Antioxidants (see Exercise and Athletic Performance)
A diet high in antioxidants may reduce the risk of many diseases (including heart disease and certain cancers). Antioxidants scavenge free radicals from the body cells and prevent or reduce the damage caused by oxidation. The protective effect of antioxidants continues to be studied around the world.

Does it work?
The broad concept behind antioxidant supplementation is relatively simple: Intense physical activity creates free radicals that damage cells and prolong recovery, and antioxidants reduce free radicals. So theoretically, consuming antioxidants like vitamin E and vitamin C should speed recovery.

Is it safe?
When taken by mouth: Antioxidants are LIKELY SAFE when taken by mouth appropriate amounts. Certain antioxidants are POSSIBLY UNSAFE when used in large doses. Antioxidants like beta-carotene and vitamin E can cause serious adverse events when used in large doses.

Apple Cider Vinegar

Apple cider vinegar, or cider vinegar, is a vinegar made from fermented apple juice, and used in salad dressings, marinades, vinaigrettes, food preservatives, and chutneys. It is made by crushing apples, then squeezing out the juice.

Does it work?
Apple cider vinegar isn't likely to be effective for weight loss. Proponents of apple cider vinegar claim that it has numerous health benefits and that drinking a small amount or taking a supplement before meals helps curb appetite and burn fat. However, there's little scientific support for these claims.

Is it safe?
Apple cider vinegar is possibly safe when used as a medicine, short-term. But it is possibly unsafe when used in large amounts, long-term. Consuming large amounts of apple cider vinegar long-term might lead to problems such as low levels of potassium. When applied to the skin: Apple cider vinegar is possibly unsafe.

Arginine (see Exercise and Athletic Performance)
Nitric oxide is a powerful neurotransmitter that helps blood vessels relax and also improves circulation. Some evidence shows that arginine may help improve blood flow in the arteries of the heart. That may improve symptoms of clogged arteries, chest pain or angina, and coronary artery disease.

Does it work?
Due to the nature of maximal incremental exercise, even a relatively small change in time to exhaustion is likely to be meaningful for athletic performance. These results suggest that L-arginine supplementation can have beneficial effects on exercise performance in elite male wrestlers.

Is it safe?
L-arginine is considered to be generally safe. It might be effective at lowering blood pressure, reducing the symptoms of angina and PAD, and treating erectile dysfunction due to a physical cause.

Ashwagandha
Ashwagandha is an evergreen shrub that grows in Asia and Africa. It is commonly used for stress. There is little evidence

for its use as an "adaptogen." Ashwagandha contains chemicals that might help calm the brain, reduce swelling, lower blood pressure, and alter the immune system.

Does it work?
Research has shown that ashwagandha can help normalize cortisol levels, thus reducing the stress response. In addition, ashwagandha has also been associated with reduced inflammation, reduced cancer risks, improved memory, improved immune function and anti-aging properties. Recent studies show that ashwagandha can increase testosterone levels in men by 10-15%, increasing strength and muscle size.

Is it safe?
When taken by mouth: Ashwagandha is possibly safe when used for up to 3 months. The long-term safety of ashwagandha is not known. Large doses of ashwagandha might cause stomach upset, diarrhea, and vomiting. Rarely, liver problems might occur.

Alpha-Ketoglutarate
α-Ketoglutaric acid is one of two ketone derivatives of glutaric acid. The term "ketoglutaric acid," when not further qualified, almost always refers to the alpha variant. β-Ketoglutaric acid varies only by the position of the ketone functional group, and is much less common.

Does it work?
Alpha-ketoglutarate is a chemical found in the body. People use it to make medicine. Alpha-ketoglutarate is used for kidney disease, intestinal and stomach disorders, and many other conditions but there is no good scientific evidence to support most of these uses.

Is it safe?
Alpha-ketoglutarate is POSSIBLY SAFE for most adults when used appropriately.

Astragalus
Astragalus propinquus, in Mongolia, is a flowering plant in the family Fabaceae. It is one of the 50 fundamental herbs used in traditional Mongolian medicine. It is a perennial plant and it is not listed as being threatened.

Does it work?
Proponents also say astragalus stimulates the spleen, liver, lungs, circulatory, and urinary system. It's also used to treat osteoarthritis, asthma, and nervous conditions as well as to lower blood sugar and blood pressure. However, there is limited evidence to prove that it is effective.

Is it safe?
When used appropriately, astragalus appears to be very safe and to have few side effects. Very high doses may suppress the immune system. So you should avoid using astragalus if you are taking immune-suppressing drugs. Pregnant or nursing women should not use astragalus root.

Vitamin A
Vitamin A is the name of a group of fat-soluble retinoids, including retinol, retinal, and retinyl esters. Vitamin A is involved in immune function, vision, reproduction, and cellular communication.

Does it work?
Vitamin A helps form and maintain healthy teeth, skeletal and soft tissue, mucus membranes, and skin. It is also known as retinol because it produces the pigments in the retina of the eye. Vitamin A promotes good eyesight, especially in low light. It also has a role in healthy pregnancy and breastfeeding.

Is it safe?
Since too much vitamin A can be harmful, consult with your doctor before taking vitamin A supplements. Vitamin A toxicity may cause symptoms, such as liver damage, vision disturbances, nausea and even death. High-dose vitamin A supplements should be avoided unless prescribed by your doctor.

Alpha-Lipoic Acid
Lipoic acid, also known as α-lipoic acid, alpha-lipoic acid and thioctic acid, is an organosulfur compound derived from caprylic acid. ALA is made in animals normally, and is essential for aerobic metabolism.

Does it work?
Alpha-lipoic acid is an organic compound with antioxidant properties. It's made in small amounts by your body but also found in foods and as a supplement. It may benefit diabetes, skin aging, memory, heart health, and weight loss. Dosages of 300–600 mg seem effective and safe without serious side effects.

Is it safe?
Alpha-lipoic acid is generally considered safe with little to no side effects. In some cases, people may experience mild symptoms like nausea, rashes, or itching. However, research shows that adults can take up to 2,400 mg without harmful side effects.

B

Bacopa Monnieri
Bacopa (Bacopa Monnieri) is a plant that has been used for centuries in traditional Ayurvedic medicine. It is sometimes called Brahmi. Bacopa might increase certain brain chemicals that are involved in thinking, learning, and memory. It might also protect brain cells from chemicals involved in Alzheimer disease.

Does it work?
In a recent study, the monnieri-treated group showed improved working memory together with a decrease in both N100 and P300 latencies. The suppression of plasma AChE activity was also observed. These results suggest that B. monnieri can improve attention, cognitive processing, and working memory partly via the suppression of AChE activity.

Is it safe?
Bacopa extract is POSSIBLY SAFE for adults when taken by mouth appropriately and short-term, up to 12 weeks. Common side effects include increased bowel movements, stomach cramps, nausea, dry mouth, and fatigue.

BCAAs (Branched-Chain Amino Acids) (see Exercise and Athletic Performance)
Studies have demonstrated that BCAAs are the key amino acids that stimulate protein synthesis (muscle building) after

intense exercise 3. They may play a key role in enhancing recovery and/or training adaptations. Therefore, BCAAs may have potential benefits for both endurance and strength/power exercise performance 5.

Does it work?
Data show that BCAA supplementation before and after exercise has beneficial effects for decreasing exercise-induced muscle damage and promoting muscle-protein synthesis.

Is it safe?
Taking BCAA supplements is generally safe and without side effects for most people. However, individuals with a rare congenital disorder called maple syrup urine disease should limit their intake of BCAAs because their bodies cannot break them down properly.

Bee Pollen
Bee pollen, also known as bee bread and ambrosia, is a ball or pellet of field-gathered flower pollen packed by worker honeybees, and used as the primary food source for the hive. It consists of simple sugars, protein, minerals and vitamins, fatty acids, and a small percentage of other components. Bee pollen is stored in brood cells, mixed with saliva, and sealed with a drop of honey. Bee pollen is harvested as food for humans and marketed as having various, but yet unproven, health benefits

Does it work?
Bee pollen contains many vitamins, minerals and antioxidants, making it incredibly healthy. Studies have linked bee pollen and its compounds to health benefits such as decreased inflammation, as well as improved immunity, menopausal symptoms and wound healing.

Is it safe?
Bee pollen is an excellent source of a wide variety of nutrients. It is generally safe for most people when taken by mouth. However, long-term use may cause serious side effects, including muscle weakness, nausea, numbness, skin rash, swelling or trouble breathing.

Beetroot (Beet Juice) (see Exercise and Athletic Performance)

The beetroot is the taproot portion of a beet plant, usually known in North America as beets while the vegetable is referred to as beetroot in British English, and also known as the table beet, garden beet, red beet, dinner beet or golden beet.

Does it work?

Beetroot contains nitrates, meaning they boost our body's levels of nitric oxide. Nitric oxide - a gas already naturally occurring in the body - tells our blood vessels to expand, increasing blood flow and lowering blood pressure.

Is it safe?

When taken by mouth: Beet is LIKELY SAFE for most people when taken in the amounts typically found in foods. Beet is POSSIBLY SAFE for most people when taken by mouth in medicinal amounts. Beet can make urine or stools appear pink or red. But this is not harmful.

Berberine

Berberine is a chemical found in some plants like European barberry, goldenseal, goldthread, Oregon grape, phellodendron, and tree turmeric. Berberine is a bitter-tasting and yellow-colored chemical. It might help strengthen the heartbeat, which could benefit people with certain heart conditions.

Does it work?

Many studies show that berberine can significantly reduce blood sugar levels in individuals with type 2 diabetes. In fact, its effectiveness is comparable to the popular diabetes drug metformin (Glucophage).

Is it safe?

When taken by mouth: Berberine is possibly safe for most adults. It's been used safely in doses up to 1.5 grams daily for 6 months. Common side effects include diarrhea, constipation, gas, and upset stomach. When applied to the skin: Berberine is possibly safe for most adults when used short-term.

Beta-alanine (see Exercise and Athletic Performance)

Beta-alanine is a non-essential amino acid that is produced naturally in the body. Beta-alanine aids in the production of carnosine. That's a compound that plays a role in muscle endurance in high-intensity exercise.

Does it work?
β-alanine supplementation has also been shown to increase resistance training performance and training volume in team-sport athletes, which may allow for greater overload and superior adaptations compared with training alone.

Is it safe?
Although excessive amounts may cause tingling in the skin, beta-alanine is considered to be a safe and effective supplement to boost exercise performance.

Beta-Carotene (see Vitamin A)
Beta Carotene is a compound that gives vivid yellow, orange, and red coloring to vegetables. The body converts Beta Carotene into vitamin A (retinol). Vitamin A, known as a vital nutrient for vision, plays a critical role in cell growth and in maintaining healthy organs like the heart, lungs, and kidneys.

Does it work?
It gives yellow and orange fruits and vegetables their rich hues. Beta-carotene is also used to color foods such as margarine. In the body, beta-carotene converts into vitamin A (retinol). We need vitamin A for good vision and eye health, for a strong immune system, and for healthy skin and mucous membranes.

Is it safe?
We need vitamin A for good vision and eye health, for a strong immune system, and for healthy skin and mucous membranes. Taking big doses of vitamin A can be toxic, but your body only converts as much vitamin A from beta-carotene as it needs. That means beta-carotene is considered a safe source of vitamin A.

Beta-Glucans (see Weight Loss)
Beta-glucans are soluble dietary fibers in bacteria, yeasts, fungi, oats, and barley. They might slow down the time it takes

for food to travel through your digestive system, making you feel fuller.

Does it work?
Beta-glucans don't seem to have any effect on body weight.

Is it safe?
Beta-glucans seem to be safe (at up to 10 grams a day for 12 weeks). They can cause flatulence.

Beta-Hydroxy-Beta-Methylbutyrate (HMB) (see Exercise and Athletic Performance)

β-Hydroxy β-methylbutyric acid (HMB), otherwise known as its conjugate base, β-hydroxy β-methylbutyrate, is a naturally produced substance in humans that is used as a dietary supplement and as an ingredient in certain medical foods that are intended to promote wound healing and provide nutritional support for people with muscle wasting due to cancer or HIV/AIDS

Does it work?
The International Society of Sports Nutrition (ISSN) bases the following on a critical analysis of the literature on the use of beta-hydroxy-beta-methylbutyrate (HMB) as a nutritional supplement. The ISSN has concluded the following: 1. HMB can be used to enhance recovery by attenuating exercise induced skeletal muscle damage in trained and untrained populations. 2. If consuming HMB, an athlete will benefit from consuming the supplement in close proximity to their workout. 3. HMB appears to be most effective when consumed for 2 weeks prior to an exercise bout. 4. Thirty-eight mg·kg·BM-1 daily of HMB has been demonstrated to enhance skeletal muscle hypertrophy, strength, and power in untrained and trained populations when the appropriate exercise prescription is utilized.

Is it safe?
beta-hydroxy-beta-methylbutyrate (HMB) supplementation in humans is safe and may decrease cardiovascular risk factors.

Betaine (see Exercise and Athletic Performance)

Betaine also called betaine anhydrous, or trimethylglycine (TMG), is a substance that's made in the body. It's involved in liver function, cellular reproduction, and helping make carnitine. It also helps the body metabolize an amino acid called homocysteine.

Does it work?
Betaine anhydrous supplements are sometimes used for reducing blood homocysteine levels, improving athletic performance, and many other purposes, but there is no good scientific evidence to support these uses.

Is it safe?
When taken by mouth: Betaine anhydrous is LIKELY SAFE for most adults. Betaine anhydrous can cause some minor side effects. These include nausea, stomach upset, and diarrhea, as well as body odor.

Bilberry
Bilberries, or occasionally European blueberries, are a primarily Eurasian species of low-growing shrubs in the genus Vaccinium, bearing edible, dark blue berries. The species most often referred to is Vaccinium myrtillus L., but there are several other closely related species.

Does it work?
Bilberry contains chemicals called tannins that can help improve diarrhea, as well as mouth and throat irritation, by reducing swelling (inflammation). There is some evidence that the chemicals found in bilberry leaves can help lower blood sugar and cholesterol levels.

Is it safe?
Bilberry fruit and extract are considered generally safe, with no known side effects. However, bilberry leaf and extract should not be taken in large quantities over an extended period of time because the tannins they contain may cause severe weight loss, muscle spasms, and even death.

Biotin
Biotin (vitamin B7) is a vitamin found in foods like eggs, milk, and bananas. Biotin deficiency can cause thinning of the hair and a rash on the face. Biotin is an important part of

enzymes in the body that break down substances like fats, carbohydrates, and others.

Does it work?

Biotin, also known as vitamin B7, stimulates keratin production in hair and can increase the rate of follicle growth. It is not stored for long in the body - most of yours is from the foods you eat. In order to be effective, it needs to be consumed. According to a 2017 review in the journal Skin Appendage Disorders, there is little conclusive evidence that biotin reduces hair loss, but it remains a popular supplement for hair, skin, and nail growth.

Is it safe?

When taken by mouth: Biotin is likely safe for most people when taken in doses up to 300 mg daily for up to 6 months. But it is more commonly used in lower doses of 2.5 mg daily. When applied to the skin: Biotin is likely safe for most people when applied in cosmetic products that contain up to 0.6% biotin.

Bitter Melon

Momordica charantia is a tropical and subtropical vine of the family Cucurbitaceae, widely grown in Asia, Africa, and the Caribbean for its edible fruit. Its many varieties differ substantially in the shape and bitterness of the fruit.

Does it work?

Bitter melon isn't an approved treatment or medication for prediabetes or diabetes despite the evidence that it can manage blood sugar. Several studies have examined bitter melon and diabetes. Most recommend conducting more research before using any form of the melon for diabetes management.

Is it safe?

At least in the short-term, bitter melon seems to be safe. It can cause headaches, upset stomach, cramping, and diarrhea. Risks. Bitter melon may affect blood sugar levels.

Bitter Orange

Bitter orange contains synephrine (a stimulant). It's claimed to burn calories, increase fat breakdown, and decrease appetite. Products with bitter orange usually also contain caffeine and other ingredients. Bitter orange is in some weight loss dietary supplements that used to contain ephedra, another stimulant-containing herb that was banned from the U.S. market in 2004 (see the section on ephedra).

Does it work?
Bitter orange might slightly increase the number of calories you burn. It might also reduce your appetite a little, but whether it can help you lose weight is unknown.

Is it safe?
Bitter orange might not be safe. Supplements with bitter orange can cause chest pain, anxiety, headache, muscle and bone pain, a faster heart rate, and higher blood pressure.

Black Cohosh
Black cohosh (Actaea racemose) is a woodland herb native to North America. The root is used as medicine and is often used for estrogen-related conditions. In some parts of the body, black cohosh might increase the effects of estrogen. In other parts of the body, black cohosh might decrease the effects of estrogen.

Does it work?
Based on current research, black cohosh is most likely to relieve symptoms related to reductions or imbalances in the hormone estrogen. A 2010 review concluded menopausal women experienced a 26 percent reduction in night sweats and hot flashes when using black cohosh supplements.

Is it safe?
In clinical trials, people have taken black cohosh for as long as 12 months with no serious harmful effects. Black cohosh can cause some mild side effects, such as stomach upset, cramping, headache, rash, a feeling of heaviness, vaginal spotting or bleeding, and weight gain.

Blessed Thistle
Cnicus benedictus, is a thistle-like plant in the family Asteraceae, native to the Mediterranean region, from Portugal north to southern France and east to Iran. It is known in other parts of the world, including parts of North America, as an introduced species and often a noxious weed.

Does it work?
Blessed thistle contains chemicals called tannins, which might help with diarrhea, cough, and swelling. People use blessed thistle for indigestion, infections, wounds, and many other conditions, but there is no good scientific evidence to support these uses. Don't confuse blessed thistle with milk thistle.

Is it safe?
Blessed thistle might be safe for most people. In high doses, such as more than 5 grams per cup of tea, blessed thistle can cause stomach irritation and vomiting.

Blue-Green Algae
blue-green algae, also called cyanobacteria, any of a large, heterogeneous group of prokaryotic, principally photosynthetic organisms.

Does it work?
Some blue-green algae can produce toxins, some do not. However, exposure to any blue-green algae blooms can cause health effects in people and animals when water with blooms is touched, swallowed, or when airborne droplets are inhaled.

Is it safe?
When taken by mouth: Blue-green algae products that are free of contaminants are possibly safe for most people when used short-term. Doses up to 19 grams daily have been used safely for up to 2 months.

Blueberry
Blueberries are a widely distributed and widespread group of perennial flowering plants with blue or purple berries. They are classified in the section Cyanococcus within the genus Vaccinium. Vaccinium also includes cranberries, bilberries, huckleberries and Madeira blueberries.

Does it work?
Blueberries are high in fiber, which can help with normal digestion. They also contain vitamin C, other antioxidants, and chemicals that might reduce swelling and destroy cancer cells.People use blueberry for aging, memory and thinking skills, high blood pressure, athletic performance, diabetes, and

many other conditions, but there is no good scientific evidence to support these uses.

Is it safe?
Blueberries are edible fruits from the Vaccinium angustifolium plant. Blueberry is a common food and is also sometimes used as medicine. Blueberries are high in fiber, which can help with normal digestion.

Boswellia Serrata
Boswellia serrata is a plant that produces Indian frankincense. It is also known as Indian oli-banum, Salai guggul, and Sallaki in Sanskrit. The plant is native to much of India and the Punjab region that extends into Pakistan.

Does it work?
Because boswellia is an effective anti-inflammatory, it can be an effective painkiller and may prevent the loss of cartilage. Some studies have found that it may even be useful in treating certain cancers, such as leukemia and breast cancer.

Is it safe?
When taken by mouth: Boswellia serrata is likely safe for most adults. Boswellia serrata extract has been used safely in doses up to 1000 mg daily for up to 6 months. It usually doesn't cause major side effects. But some people have reported stomach pain, nausea, diarrhea, heartburn, and itching.

Bone Meal
Bone meal is a mixture of finely and coarsely ground animal bones and slaughter-house waste products. It is used as a dietary supplement to supply calcium (Ca) and phosphorus (P) to monogastric livestock. As an slow-release organic fertilizer, it supplies P, Ca, and a small amount of N to plants.

Does it work?
Bone meal can increase soil microbes throughout the growing season, benefitting the soil structure for the root systems of your plants. Bone meal provides calcium for your plants. Calcium improves root growth, encourages strong

roots, and helps prevent blossom end rot. Bone meal can balance other soil amendments.

Is it safe?
There are no studies that show if bone meal is safe for human consumption. There are no known significant food or medicine interactions with bone meal.

Boron
Boron is an element. Boron has been consumed for menstrual cramps and boric acid has been used vaginally for yeast infections, but evidence is limited. Boron seems to affect the way the body handles other minerals such as calcium, magnesium, and phosphorus. It also seems to increase estrogen levels post-menopause.

Does it work?
As the current article shows, boron has been proven to be an important trace mineral because it is essential for the growth and maintenance of bone; greatly improves wound healing; beneficially impacts the body's use of estrogen, testosterone, and vitamin D; boosts magnesium absorption

Is it safe?
Boron is possibly unsafe when taken in higher doses. Doses over 20 mg daily might cause male fertility problems. Large doses can also cause poisoning. Signs of poisoning include irritability, tremors, weakness, headaches, diarrhea, vomiting, and other symptoms

Botanical Dietary Supplements
A dietary supplement is a manufactured product intended to supplement one's diet by taking a pill, capsule, tablet, powder, or liquid. A supplement can provide nutrients either extracted from food sources or that are synthetic in order to increase the quantity of their consumption.

Does it work?
While dietary supplements cannot take the place of healthy eating habits, they can provide adequate amounts of essential nutrients when used responsibly.Maintain their general

health.Maintain their general health.Support mental and sports-related performance.Provide immune system support.

Is it safe?

The actions of botanicals range from mild to powerful. A botanical with mild action might have subtle effects. Chamomile and peppermint, for example, are usually consumed in teas to help with digestion and are generally considered safe for most people. Some botanicals with mild action might need to be taken for weeks or months before their full effects are achieved. For example, valerian might help users sleep better after a few weeks of use, but just one dose is rarely effective. In contrast, a powerful botanical produces a fast result. Green tea (a natural source of caffeine) and yohimbe, for example, can have strong and immediate stimulant effects.

Branched-chain amino acids (see Exercise and Athletic Performance)

Branched-chain amino acids (BCAAs) are essential nutrients including leucine, isoleucine, and valine. They're found in meat, dairy, and legumes. BCAAs stimulate the building of protein in muscle and possibly reduce muscle breakdown. The "Branched-chain" refers to the chemical structure of these amino acids.

Does it work?

Branched-chain amino acids (BCAAs; valine, leucine, and isoleucine) are essential amino acids with protein anabolic properties, which have been studied in a number of muscle wasting disorders for more than 50 years. However, until today, there is no consensus regarding their therapeutic effectiveness.

Is it safe?

When taken by mouth: BCAAs are likely safe when used in doses of 12 grams daily for up to 2 years. It might cause some side effects, such as fatigue and loss of coordination. BCAAs should be used cautiously before or during activities that require motor coordination, such as driving.

Bromelain

Bromelain is a type of enzyme called a proteolytic enzyme. It is found in pineapple juice and in the pineapple stem. Bromelain causes the body to make substances that fight pain and swelling. Bromelain also contains chemicals that seem to interfere with tumor cells and slow blood clotting.

Does it work?
A review of clinical studies found that bromelain's anti-inflammatory and analgesic properties make it an effective treatment for the pain, soft-tissue swelling, and joint stiffness associated with osteoarthritis.

Is it safe?
When taken by mouth: Bromelain is possibly safe for most people. Doses of up to 240 mg daily have been used safely for up to one year. Bromelain might cause some side effects, including diarrhea and stomach upset. When applied to the skin: Bromelain is possibly safe.

Bentonite Clay
Bentonite is a very old clay that has been used as a remedy for many things. The fine powder forms when volcanic ash ages. It's named after Fort Benton, WY, which has a lot of it. But it's found all over the world. It's also known as Montmorillonite clay after a region in France with a large deposit.

Does it work?
According to some research, bentonite clay may be helpful in removing some lead from the body. Bentonite clay has a negative charge, meaning that it can bind to positively charged metals such as lead. One study found that bentonite clay was effective at removing lead from wastewater.

Is it safe?
Bentonite clay is generally OK to use on your skin and hair. But the FDA doesn't regulate health and cosmetic products, so there's no way to know exactly what's in them or if they'll work. If you want to try it, test a little bit of the clay on your skin first to make sure you don't have a bad reaction.

Butterbur

Butterbur is a shrub that grows in Europe and parts of Asia and North America. The name, butterbur, is attributed to the traditional use of its large leaves to wrap butter in warm weather.

Does it work?
Some studies of butterbur root or leaf extracts suggest that they may be helpful for symptoms of hay fever (allergic rhinitis), but the data are not convincing. One study suggested that a combination product containing butterbur might improve anxiety and depression in people with somatoform disorders.

Is it safe?
Some butterbur products contain chemicals called pyrrolizidine alkaloids (PAs). PAs can damage the liver, lungs, and blood circulation, and possibly cause cancer. Only butterbur products that have been processed to remove PAs and are labeled or certified as PA-free should be considered for use.

Vitamin B1 (see Thiamin)
Thiamine, also known as thiamin and vitamin B_1, is a vitamin, an essential micronutrient, which cannot be made in the body. It is found in food and commercially synthesized to be a dietary supplement or medication. Food sources of thiamine include whole grains, legumes, and some meats and fish.

Does it work?
A dose of vitamins B1 and B12 can help improve nerve pain in people with diabetes and may reduce the need for painkillers. Improves memory. Getting enough thiamine can help improve concentration and memory. Because of its positive effect on attitude and brain function, it is also known as a "morale vitamin".

Is it safe?
Thiamine is generally safe. Very high doses may cause stomach upset. Taking any one of the B vitamins for a long period of time can result in an imbalance of other important B vitamins.

Vitamin B12

Vitamin B12 is a nutrient that helps keep your body's blood and nerve cells healthy and helps make DNA, the genetic material in all of your cells. Vitamin B12 also helps prevent megaloblastic anemia, a blood condition that makes people tired and weak.

Does it work?

Vitamin B12 is needed to form red blood cells and DNA. It is also a key player in the function and development of brain and nerve cells. Vitamin B12 binds to the protein in the foods we eat. In the stomach, hydrochloric acid and enzymes unbind vitamin B12 into its free form.

Is it safe?

When taken at appropriate doses, vitamin B-12 supplements are generally considered safe. While the recommended daily amount of vitamin B-12 for adults is 2.4 micrograms, higher doses have been found to be safe. Your body absorbs only as much as it needs, and any excess passes through your urine.

Vitamin B2 (see Riboflavin)

Riboflavin, also known as vitamin B_2, is a vitamin found in food and sold as a dietary supplement. It is essential to the formation of two major coenzymes, flavin mononucleotide and flavin adenine dinucleotide.

Does it work?

Riboflavin (vitamin B2) works with the other B vitamins. It is important for body growth. It helps in red blood cell production. It also aids in the release of energy from proteins.

Is it safe?

Normally, vitamin B2 is considered safe. An overdose is unlikely, as the body can absorb up to around 27 milligrams of riboflavin, and it expels any additional amounts in the urine. However, it is important to talk to a physician before taking any supplements, especially as these can interfere with other medications.

Vitamin B Complex

Vitamin B complex is composed of eight B vitamins:

B-1 (thiamine), B-2 (riboflavin), B-3 (niacin), B-5 (pantothenic acid), B-6 (pyridoxine)

B-7 (biotin), B-9 (folic acid), B-12 (cobalamin)

Does it work?
B vitamins play a vital role in maintaining good health and well-being. As the building blocks of a healthy body, B vitamins have a direct impact on your energy levels, brain function, and cell metabolism.

Is it safe?
Although taking a vitamin B complex as directed is likely safe, consuming high doses of B3 or B6 can lead to serious side effects.

Vitamin B3 (see Niacin)
Niacin is a form of vitamin B3 made in the body from tryptophan. It's found in many foods including meat, fish, milk, eggs, green vegetables, and cereals. Niacin is required for the proper function of fats and sugars in the body and to maintain healthy cells.

Does it work?
Niacin is an important nutrient. In fact, every part of your body needs it to function properly. As a supplement, niacin may help lower cholesterol, ease arthritis, and boost brain function, among other benefits.

Is it safe?
At the low DRI doses, niacin is safe for everyone. However, at the higher amounts used to treat medical conditions, it can have risks. For that reason, children and women who are pregnant or breastfeeding should not take niacin supplements in excess of the DRI unless it's recommended by a doctor.

Vitamin B5 (see Pantothenic Acid)
Pantothenic acid, also called vitamin B_5 is a water-soluble B vitamin and therefore an essential nutrient. All animals require pantothenic acid in order to synthesize coenzyme A essential for fatty acid metabolism as well as to, in general, synthesize and metabolize proteins, carbohydrates, and fats.

Does it work?

In addition to playing a role in the breakdown of fats and carbohydrategls for energy, vitamin B5 is critical to the manufacture of red blood cells, as well as sex and stress-related hormones produced in the adrenal glands, small glands that sit atop the kidneys.

Is it safe?
Doctors consider vitamin B5 safe at doses equal to the daily intake, and at moderately higher doses. Very high doses may cause diarrhea and may increase the risk of bleeding. Pregnant and breastfeeding women should not exceed the daily adequate intake unless directed by their doctor.

Vitamin B6
Vitamin B_6 is one of the B vitamins, and thus an essential nutrient. The term refers to a group of six chemically similar compounds, i.e., "vitamers", which can be interconverted in biological systems.

Does it work?
Vitamin B6 helps maintain a normal amount of this amino acid in your blood. A stronger immune system. Vitamin B6 helps chemical reactions in the immune system, helping it work better. Eating foods rich in vitamin B6 will help your body guard against infection.

Is it safe?
Taking vitamin B6 in doses of 100 mg daily or less is generally considered to be safe. Vitamin B6 is possibly safe when taken in doses of 101-200 mg daily. In some people, vitamin B6 might cause nausea, stomach pain, loss of appetite, headache, and other side effects.

Vitamin B7 (see Biotin)
Biotin, also called vitamin B_7, is one of the B vitamins. It is involved in a wide range of metabolic processes, both in humans and in other organisms, primarily related to the utilization of fats, carbohydrates, and amino acids. The name biotin derives from the Greek word "bios" and the suffix "-in".

Does it work?
Biotin supplements are often glamorized as a treatment for hair loss and to promote healthy hair, skin, and nails.

Although a deficiency of biotin can certainly lead to hair loss and skin or nail problems, evidence showing a benefit of supplementation is inconclusive.

Is it safe?
When taken by mouth: Biotin is likely safe for most people when taken in doses up to 300 mg daily for up to 6 months. But it is more commonly used in lower doses of 2.5 mg daily. When applied to the skin: Biotin is likely safe for most people when applied in cosmetic products that contain up to 0.6% biotin.

Beta-Sitosterol
β-sitosterol is one of several phytosterols with chemical structures similar to that of cholesterol. It is a white, waxy powder with a characteristic odor, and is one of the components of the food additive E499. Phytosterols are hydrophobic and soluble in alcohols.

Does it work?
Taking 60-130 mg of beta-sitosterol by mouth in divided doses daily helps improve symptoms of BPH. But it doesn't actually shrink an enlarged prostate. High cholesterol. Taking beta-sitosterol by mouth can lower total and low-density lipoprotein (LDL or "bad") cholesterol levels.

Is it safe?
When taken by mouth: Beta-sitosterol is likely safe for most people. It's been used safely at a dose of up to 20 grams daily for up to 3 months. It's also been used at a lower dose of 130 mg daily for up to 18 months. It can cause some mild side effects, such as nausea, indigestion, gas, diarrhea, or constipation.

Vitamin B9 (see Folate)
Folate, also known as vitamin B_9 and folacin, is one of the B vitamins. Manufactured folic acid, which is converted into folate by the body, is used as a dietary supplement and in food fortification as it is more stable during processing and storage.

Does it work?
It aids in the production of DNA and RNA, the body's genetic material, and is especially important when cells and

tissues are growing rapidly, such as in infancy, adolescence, and pregnancy. Folic acid also works closely with vitamin B12 to help make red blood cells and help iron work properly in the body.

Is it safe?
Toxicity. It is extremely rare to reach a toxic level when eating folate from food sources. However, an upper limit for folic acid is set at 1,000 mcg daily because studies have shown that taking higher amounts can mask a vitamin B12 deficiency.

C

Caffeine
Caffeine is a stimulant that can make you more alert, give you a boost of energy, burn calories, and increase fat breakdown. Often added to weight-loss dietary supplements, caffeine is found naturally in tea, guarana, kola (cola) nut, yerba mate, and other herbs. The labels of supplements that contain caffeine don't always list it, so you might not know if a supplement has caffeine.

Does it work?
Weight-loss dietary supplements with caffeine might help you lose a little weight or gain less weight over time. But when you use caffeine regularly, you become tolerant of it. This tolerance might lessen any effect of caffeine on body weight over time.

Is it safe?
Caffeine is safe for most adults at doses up to 400–500 milligrams (mg) a day. But it can make you feel nervous, jittery, and shaky. It can also affect your sleep. At higher doses, it can cause nausea, vomiting, rapid heartbeat, and seizures. Combining caffeine with other stimulant ingredients can increase caffeine's effects.

Collagen
Collagen is the main structural protein in the extracellular matrix found in the body's various connective tissues. As the main component of connective tissue, it is the most abundant

protein in mammals, making up from 25% to 35% of the whole-body protein content.

Does it work?
The scientific evidence for using collagen supplements to reduce wrinkles and relieving joint pain associated with osteoarthritis is promising, but higher quality studies are needed. Collagen supplements have not been studied much for muscle building, improving bone density, and other benefits.

Is it safe?
When taken by mouth: Collagen peptides are possibly safe. Collagen peptides have been safely used in doses up to 10 grams daily for up to 5 months. Side effects are rare.

Curcumin
Curcumin is a bright yellow chemical produced by plants of the Curcuma longa species. It is the principal curcuminoid of turmeric (Curcuma longa), a member of the ginger family, Zingiberaceae. It is sold as an herbal supplement, cosmetics ingredient, food flavoring, and food coloring.

Does it work?
The main active ingredient found in turmeric is curcumin. Curcumin is an inflammation blocker. It's as effective as some anti-inflammatory drugs without the major side effects. That's a big deal because inflammation plays a role in every major disease.

Is it safe?
Turmeric and curcumin are considered safe for most people. There are few if any reports of people experiencing negative reactions to typical amounts of turmeric in food, and curcumin supplements are generally well tolerated. Taking curcumin supplements may suppress iron absorption.

Calcium
Calcium is a mineral you need for healthy bones, muscles, nerves, blood vessels, and many of your body's functions. It's claimed to burn fat and decrease fat absorption.

Does it work?

Calcium either from food or in weight-loss dietary supplements probably doesn't help you lose weight or prevent weight gain.

Is it safe?

Calcium is safe at the recommended amounts of 1,000 to 1,200 mg a day for adults. Too much calcium (more than 2,000–2,500 mg a day) can cause constipation and decrease your body's absorption of iron and zinc. Also, too much calcium from supplements (but not foods) might increase your risk of kidney stones.

Calendula

Calendula is a genus of about 15–20 species of annual and perennial herbaceous plants in the daisy family Asteraceae that are often known as marigolds. They are native to southwestern Asia, western Europe, Macaronesia, and the Mediterranean.

Does it work?

Calendula has been used to treat a variety of ailments affecting the skin as well as infections and fungus. Research suggests that calendula may be effective in treating diaper rash, wounds, vaginal yeast infections, and other skin conditions. Calendula has also been used as a pain reducer and inflammation reducer.

Is it safe?

Calendula is generally considered safe to use on your skin. Do not apply it to an open wound without a doctor's supervision. People who are allergic to plants in the daisy or aster family, including chrysanthemums and ragweed, may also have an allergic reaction to calendula (usually a skin rash).

Cannabidiol (CBD)

Cannabidiol (CBD) is a chemical in the Cannabis sativa plant, also known as cannabis or hemp. One specific form of CBD is approved as a drug in the U.S. for seizure. Over 80 chemicals, known as cannabinoids, have been found in the Cannabis sativa plant.

Does it work?

There is moderate evidence that CBD can improve sleep disorders, fibromyalgia pain, muscle spasticity related to multiple sclerosis, and anxiety. People report that oral CBD helps relieve anxiety and pain and also leads to better sleep.

Is it safe?
Though it's often well-tolerated, CBD can cause side effects, such as dry mouth, diarrhea, reduced appetite, drowsiness and fatigue. CBD can also interact with other medications you're taking, such as blood thinners.

Capsaicin (see Weight Loss)
Capsaicin comes from chili peppers and makes them taste hot. It's claimed to help burn fat and calories and to help you feel full and eat less.

Does it work?
Capsaicin hasn't been studied enough to know if it will help you lose weight.

Is it safe?
Capsaicin is safe (at up to 33 mg a day for 4 weeks or 4 mg a day for 12 weeks), but it can cause stomach pain, burning sensations, nausea, and bloating.

Crocin
Crocin is a carotenoid chemical compound that is found in the flowers crocus and gardenia. Crocin is the chemical primarily responsible for the color of saffron. Chemically, crocin is the diester formed from the disaccharide gentiobiose and the dicarboxylic acid crocetin.

Does it work?
It functions by blocking the release of certain chemicals that are responsible for pain and fever. A popular painkiller used for the treatment of aches and pains is Crocin Advance Tablet. It works by suppressing the brain's chemical messengers that tell us we're in pain.

Is it safe?
Crocin medication is commonly used and considered safe, but it is not sufficient for all. Before taking this drug, let your doctor know if you have problems with your liver or kidneys, or

if you are using blood thinners. The dosage or suitability of this drug can be influenced by it.

Capsaicinoids

Capsaicinoids are the name given to the class of compounds found in members of the capsicum family (also known as peppers). The most common capsaicinoid is capsaicin. Capsaicin, is the chemical compound that gives hot chile peppers the heat you experience when eating them.

Does it work?

Capsaicin is taken from chilli peppers. It works mainly by reducing Substance P, a pain transmitter in your nerves. Results from RCTs assessing its role in treating osteoarthritis suggest that it can be effective in reducing pain and tenderness in affected joints, and it has no major safety problems.

Is it safe?

Is it safe? There are no major safety concerns in applying capsaicin gel/cream. You may feel a burning sensation when the gel touches your skin. This is because capsaicin also binds to specific receptors in nerve endings called VR1, producing a burning sensation which isn't caused by any tissue damage.

Capsicum

Capsicum, also known as red pepper or chili pepper, is an herb. Its fruit is commonly applied to the skin for arthritis pain and other conditions. The fruit of the capsicum plant contains a chemical called capsaicin. Capsaicin is what seems to help reduce pain and swelling.

Does it work?

Capsicum is commonly used for nerve pain and other painful conditions. It is also used for many other purposes, including digestion problems, conditions of the heart and blood vessels, and many others, but there is no good scientific evidence for many of these uses.

Is it safe?

When taken by mouth: Capsicum is likely safe when consumed in amounts typically found in food. Capsaicin, the active chemical in capsicum, is possibly safe when used short-term. Side effects can include stomach irritation, sweating, and runny nose.

Carnitine
Your body makes carnitine, and it's also found in meat, fish, poultry, milk, and dairy products. In your cells, it helps break down fats.

Does it work?
Carnitine supplements might help you lose a small amount of weight.

Is it safe?
Carnitine supplements seem to be safe (at up to 2 g a day for 1 year or 4 g a day for 56 days). They can cause nausea, vomiting, diarrhea, abdominal cramps, and a fishy body odor.

Cartilage (Bovine and Shark)
Cartilage is a non-vascular type of supporting connective tissue that is found throughout the body . Cartilage is a flexible connective tissue that differs from bone in several ways; it is avascular and its microarchitecture is less organized than bone.

Does it work?
Hyaline, or articular, cartilage covers the ends of bones to create a low-friction environment and cushion at the joint surface. When cartilage in the joint is healthy, it effectively allows fluid bending/straightening motions and protects the joint against weight-bearing stresses.

Is it safe?
This is because, without proper sterile precautions and other safety measures, cartilage piercings carry a high risk of infections at the pierced area, which can delay the healing.

Cascara Sagrada
Frangula purshiana is a species of plant in the family Rhamnaceae. It is native to western North America from southern British Columbia south to central California, and eastward to northwestern Montana.

Does it work?

Cascara sagrada is a stimulant laxative. It works by causing muscle contractions in the intestines. These muscle contractions help move stool through the bowels. The bark contains chemicals called anthraquinones that give it its color and its laxative effect.

Is it safe?
When taken by mouth: Cascara sagrada is possibly safe when used for less than one week. Side effects include stomach discomfort and cramps. But cascara sagrada is possibly unsafe when used for more than one week.

Cat's Claw
Cat's claw is a woody vine that grows wild in the Amazon rainforest and other tropical areas of Central and South America. Its thorns resemble a cat's claws. The two most common species are U. tomentosa and U. guianensis.

Does it work?
Some studies suggest that cat's claw can help relieve its symptoms. For example, a study in 40 people with rheumatoid arthritis determined that 60 mg of cat's claw extract per day alongside regular medication resulted in a 29% reduction in the number of painful joints compared to a control group.

Is it safe?
While side effects of cat's claw are rarely reported, available information to determine its overall safety is currently insufficient. The high levels of tannins in cat's claw may cause some side effects — including nausea, stomach upset, and diarrhea — if consumed in large amounts.

CBD (cannabidiol)
Cannabidiol is a phytocannabinoid discovered in 1940. It is one of 113 identified cannabinoids in cannabis plants, along with tetrahydrocannabinol, and accounts for up to 40% of the plant's extract.

Does it work?
There is moderate evidence that CBD can improve sleep disorders, fibromyalgia pain, muscle spasticity related to multiple sclerosis, and anxiety. People report that oral CBD helps relieve anxiety and pain and also leads to better sleep.

Is it safe?
Although CBD is generally considered safe, it can cause adverse effects such as diarrhea and fatigue in some people. It may also interact with certain medications, causing side effects that may be harmful.

Cesium
Caesium is a chemical element with the symbol Cs and atomic number 55. It is a soft, silvery-golden alkali metal with a melting point of 28.5 °C, which makes it one of only five elemental metals that are liquid at or near room temperature.

Does it work?
Cesium is incredibly accurate at timekeeping and is used in atomic clocks. The official definition of a second is the time it takes for the cesium atom to vibrate 9,192,631,770 times between energy levels. Cesium-based atomic clocks lose one second per 100 million years.

Is it safe?
Exposure to large amounts of radioactive cesium can damage cells in your body from the radiation. You might also experience acute radiation syndrome, which includes nausea, vomiting, diarrhea, bleeding, coma, and even death in cases of very high exposures.

Chamomile
Chamomile is one of the most ancient medicinal herbs known to mankind. It is a member of Asteraceae/Compositae family and represented by two common varieties viz. German Chamomile (Chamomilla recutita) and Roman Chamomile (Chamaemelum nobile).

Does it work?
Chamomile is widely regarded as a mild tranquillizer and sleep-inducer. Sedative effects may be due to the flavonoid, apigenin that binds to benzodiazepine receptors in the brain. Studies in preclinical models have shown anticonvulsant and CNS depressant effects respectively.

Is it safe?
Chamomile is likely safe when used in amounts commonly found in teas. It might be safe when used orally for medicinal

purposes over the short term. The long-term safety of using chamomile on the skin for medicinal purposes is unknown. Side effects are uncommon and may include nausea, dizziness, and allergic reactions.

Chamomile (Roman)
Chamaemelum nobile, commonly known as chamomile, is a low perennial plant found in dry fields and around gardens and cultivated grounds in Europe, North America, and South America.

Does it work?
Extracts or dried flowers of Chamaemelum nobile are used in hair care and skincare products. The plant may be used to flavor foods, in herbal teas, perfumes, and cosmetics. It is used in aromatherapy in the belief it is a calming agent to reduce stress and promote sleep.

Is it safe?
Roman chamomile is likely safe for most people when used in amounts normally found in foods. It is possibly safe when used in large amounts and, in some people, may cause vomiting. The essential oil of Roman chamomile is possibly safe when inhaled or applied to the skin.

Chasteberry
The chasteberry plant, also called chaste tree, is native to the Mediterranean region and Asia. The name "chasteberry" may reflect the traditional belief that the plant promoted chastity. Monks in the Middle Ages reportedly used it to decrease sexual desire.

Does it work?
Chasteberry is used widely to treat infertility and premenstrual syndrome (PMS). Lab studies show chasteberry contains substances that can prompt hormonal changes in the body. Various studies in humans suggest chasteberry can help reduce breast pain and other PMS symptoms, but not menopause symptoms.

Is it safe?
When used in limited amounts, chasteberry appears to be generally well tolerated. Side effects are generally mild, and

may include nausea, headache, gastrointestinal disturbances, or itching. Taking chasteberry during pregnancy or while breastfeeding may not be safe.

Chitosan (see Weight Loss)

Chitosan comes from the shells of crabs, shrimp, and lobsters. It's claimed to bind fat in the digestive tract so that your body can't absorb it.

Does it work?

Chitosan binds only a tiny amount of fat, not enough to help you lose much weight.

Is it safe?

Chitosan seems to be safe (at up to 15 g a day for 6 months). But it can cause flatulence, bloating, mild nausea, constipation, indigestion, and heartburn. If you're allergic to shellfish, you could have an allergic reaction to chitosan.

Choline

Choline is a nutrient similar to B vitamins. It can be made in the liver. It is also found in foods such as meats, fish, nuts, beans, vegetables, and eggs. Choline is used in many chemical reactions in the body. It's important in the nervous system and for the development of normal brain functioning.

Does it work?

Current scientific studies suggest that choline may improve memory and cognition and reduce the risk of ischemic stroke. Choline supports brain development and growth in newborn babies. Research also suggests that choline may reduce the risk of preeclampsia and congenital irregularities.

Is it safe?

Can choline be harmful? Getting too much choline can cause a fishy body odor, vomiting, heavy sweating and salivation, low blood pressure, and liver damage. Some research also suggests that high amounts of choline may increase the risk of heart disease.

Chondroitin

Chondroitin sulfate is a sulfated glycosaminoglycan composed of a chain of alternating sugars. It is usually found attached to proteins as part of a proteoglycan. A chondroitin chain can have over 100 individual sugars, each of which can be sulfated in variable positions and quantities.

Does it work?

The evidence that chondroitin helps with osteoarthritis is mixed. A number of studies seemed to show that it is effective. Researchers found that chondroitin appeared to reduce pain, increase joint mobility, and decrease the need for painkillers.

Is it safe?

Chondroitin seems to be safe for most people. Side effects are rare. Some people have reported headaches, mood changes, rash, hives, diarrhea, and other symptoms. If you have any side effects, stop taking the supplement and see a doctor.

Chromium

Chromium is a mineral that you need to regulate your blood sugar levels. It's claimed to increase muscle mass and fat loss and decrease appetite and food intake.

Does it work?

Chromium might help you lose a very small amount of weight and body fat.

Is it safe?

Chromium in food and supplements is safe at recommended amounts, which range from 20 to 45 micrograms a day for adults. In larger amounts, chromium can cause watery stools, headache, weakness, nausea, vomiting, constipation, dizziness, and hives.

Cinnamon

Cinnamon is a spice that is made from the inner bark of trees scientifically known as Cinnamomum. It has been used as an ingredient throughout history, dating back as far as Ancient Egypt. It used to be rare and valuable and was regarded as a gift fit for kings.

Does it work?

Cinnamon Lowers Blood Sugar Levels and Has a Powerful Anti-Diabetic Effect. Cinnamon is well known for its blood-sugar-lowering properties. Apart from the beneficial effects on insulin resistance, cinnamon can lower blood sugar by several other mechanisms.

Is it safe?
Cinnamon is generally safe to use in small amounts as a spice. It's linked to many impressive health benefits. However, eating too much may cause potentially dangerous side effects. This mostly applies to Cassia cinnamon because it's a rich source of coumarin.

Citrulline (see Exercise and Athletic Performance)
Overview. L-citrulline is an amino acid found in watermelon. It is also made in the body. The body changes L-citrulline into another amino acid called L-arginine. The name citrulline comes from Citrullus vulgaris, the Latin term for watermelon.

Does it work?
L-citrulline supplements may ease symptoms of mild-to-moderate erectile dysfunction (ED). Scientists say L-citrulline does not work as well as ED drugs such as Viagra. However, it appears to be a safe option.

Is it safe?
Citrulline is an amino acid with several health benefits. It also appears to be safe and there are currently no known side effects. This supplement may promote healthier blood vessels and lower blood pressure, especially in people with heart conditions or high blood pressure.

Chinese Herbal Medicines (CHM)
Chinese herbal medicines (CHM) and Chinese proprietary medicines (CPM) are widely used by people of Chinese origin throughout the world. Although the use of these medicinal materials rarely causes significant toxic effects, cases of severe and even fatal poisoning have occurred after medication with herbs containing aconitine, podophyllin, and anticholinergic substances.

Does it work?
Some psychological and/or physical approaches used in traditional Chinese medicine practices, such as acupuncture and tai chi, may help improve quality of life and certain pain

conditions. Studies of Chinese herbal products used in traditional Chinese medicine for a range of medical conditions have had mixed results.

Is it safe?
Some Chinese herbal products have been contaminated with toxic compounds, heavy metals, pesticides, and microorganisms and may have serious side effects. Manufacturing errors, in which one herb is mistakenly replaced with another, also have resulted in serious complications.

Clove
Clove (Syzygium aromaticum) is a tree native to Indonesia. Its dried flower buds are a popular spice and are also used in Chinese and Ayurvedic medicine. Clove oils, dried flower buds, leaves, and stems are used to make medicine.

Does it work?
Clove is also a popular ingredient in cigarettes. People commonly use clove for toothache, pain during dental work, dental plaque, hangover, indigestion, and many other conditions, but there is no good scientific evidence to support these uses.

Is it safe?
Stay on the safe side and stick to food amounts. Children: Clove oil is likely unsafe to take by mouth. Even small amounts of clove oil can cause severe side effects such as seizures, liver damage, and fluid imbalances. Bleeding disorders: Clove oil contains a chemical called eugenol that seems to slow blood clotting.

Cobalamin (see Vitamin B12)
A nutrient in the vitamin B complex that the body needs in small amounts to function and stay healthy. Cobalamin helps make red blood cells, DNA, RNA, energy, and tissues, and keeps nerve cells healthy.

Does it work?
Vitamin B12, or cobalamin, is naturally found in animal foods. It can also be added to foods or supplements. Vitamin

B12 is needed to form red blood cells and DNA. It is also a key player in the function and development of brain and nerve cells

Is it safe?

Answer: The most common form of vitamin B-12 (cobalamin) in supplements is cyanocobalamin and although this form includes a cyanide molecule, it is very safe. Why? Even at a very high dose, it would provide about a thousand times less cyanide than is toxic, and the cyanide is excreted in the urine.

Cod Liver Oil

Cod liver oil is a dietary supplement derived from liver of cod fish (Gadidae). As with most fish oils, it contains the omega-3 fatty acids eicosapentaenoic acid (EPA) and docosahexaenoic acid (DHA), and also vitamin A and vitamin D. Historically, it was given to children because vitamin D had been shown to prevent rickets, a consequence of vitamin D deficiency.

Does it work?

Cod liver oil is a good source of the omega-3 fatty acid known as docosahexaenoic acid (DHA). Studies have shown that DHA improves cognitive function and can protect against Alzheimer's disease and dementia.

Is it safe?

When taken by mouth: Cod liver oil is likely safe for most adults. It can cause side effects including heartburn, stomach upset, and nausea. High doses of cod liver oil are possibly unsafe. They might keep blood from clotting and can increase the chance of bleeding.

Coenzyme Q10

Coenzyme: A substance that enhances the action of an enzyme. (An enzyme is a protein that functions as a catalyst to mediate and speed a chemical reaction). Coenzymes are small molecules. They cannot by themselves catalyze a reaction but they can help enzymes to do so.

Does it work?

Without coenzymes or cofactors, enzymes cannot catalyze reactions effectively. In fact, the enzyme may not function at all. If reactions cannot occur at the normal catalyzed rate, then an organism will have difficulty sustaining life. When an enzyme gains a coenzyme, it then becomes a holoenzyme, or active enzyme.

Is it safe?

When taken by mouth: Coenzyme Q10 is likely safe for most adults. While most people tolerate coenzyme Q10 well, it can cause some mild side effects including stomach upset, loss of appetite, nausea, vomiting, and diarrhea.

Cola Nut (Kola Nut) (see Weight Loss)

The kola nut is the fruit of the kola tree (Cola acuminata and Cola nitida), indigenous to West Africa. The trees, which reach heights of 40 to 60 feet, produce a star-shaped fruit. Each fruit contains between two and five kola nuts. About the size of a chestnut, this little fruit is packed with caffeine.

Does it work?

Cola nut contains caffeine. Caffeine works by stimulating the central nervous system (CNS), heart, and muscles.

Is it safe?

Cola nut is possibly safe when taken by mouth in medicinal amounts, short-term. The caffeine in cola nut can cause insomnia, nervousness and restlessness, stomach irritation, nausea and vomiting, increased heart rate and respiration, and other side effects.

Coleus Forskohlii (Forskolin) (see Weight Loss)

Coleus forskohlii is a plant that grows in India, Thailand, and other subtropical areas. Forskolin, made from the plant's roots, is claimed to help you lose weight by decreasing your appetite and increasing the breakdown of fat in your body.

Does it work?

Forskolin hasn't been studied much. But so far, it doesn't seem to have any effect on body weight or appetite.

Is it safe?

Forskolin seems to be safe (at 500 mg a day for 12 weeks), but it hasn't been well studied. It can cause frequent bowel movements and loose stools.

Colloidal Silver

Colloidal silver consists of tiny silver particles in a liquid that is sometimes promoted on the Internet as a dietary supplement. However, evidence supporting health-related claims is lacking. In fact, colloidal silver can be dangerous to your health.

Does it work?

Is Colloidal Silver Effective? Scientific evidence doesn't support the use of colloidal silver dietary supplements for any disease or condition. Silver has no known function or benefits in the body when taken by mouth. Silver is not a nutritionally essential mineral or a useful dietary supplement.

Is it safe?

Is Colloidal Silver Effective? Scientific evidence doesn't support the use of colloidal silver dietary supplements for any disease or condition. Silver has no known function or benefits in the body when taken by mouth. Silver is not a nutritionally essential mineral or a useful dietary supplement.

Conjugated Linoleic Acid (see Weight Loss)

CLA is a fat found mainly in dairy products and beef. It's claimed to reduce your body fat.

Does it work?

CLA may help you lose a very small amount of weight and body fat.

Is it safe?

CLA seems to be safe (at up to 6 g a day for 1 year). It can cause an upset stomach, constipation, diarrhea, loose stools, and indigestion.

Copper

Copper is a chemical element with the symbol Cu (from Latin: cuprum) and atomic number 29. It is a soft, malleable, and ductile metal with very high thermal and electrical conductivity.

Does it work?

Studies confirm these treatments are ineffective for arthritis pain. Magnet therapy or wearing copper jewelry may seem attractive for easing your arthritis pain simply and inexpensively. But studies confirm these treatments are ineffective for arthritis pain.

Is it safe?
When taken by mouth: Copper is likely safe when used in amounts no greater than 10 mg daily. Copper is possibly unsafe when taken in larger amounts. Kidney failure and death can occur with as little as 1 gram of copper sulfate.

COVID-19
Coronavirus disease (COVID-19) is an infectious disease caused by the SARS-CoV-2 virus. Most people who fall sick with COVID-19 will experience mild to moderate symptoms and recover without special treatment. However, some will become seriously ill and require medical attention.

How it spreads?
The virus can spread from an infected person's mouth or nose in small liquid particles when they cough, sneeze, speak, sing or breathe. These particles range from larger respiratory droplets to smaller aerosols.

Cranberry
Cranberry (Vaccinium macrocarpon) is an evergreen shrub that grows in bogs in North America. It produces dark red fruits that contain salicylic acid. Chemicals in cranberries keep bacteria from sticking to the cells in the urinary tract.

Does it work?
Some studies have found that drinking cranberry juice or taking cranberry pills can prevent UTIs, especially in women who are at risk for these infections. But others haven't come to that conclusion. Cranberries don't seem to work for everyone. And they don't treat UTIs that you already have.

Is it safe?
Cranberry products are generally thought to be safe. However, if consumed in very large amounts, they can cause stomach upset and diarrhea, particularly in young children.

Comfrey Extract Gel
Comfrey cream is a natural substance made from Symphytum officinale , an herb in the borage family. Also known as comfrey ointment, salve, or gel, it's said to reduce

inflammation (swelling) and alleviate pain when applied to the skin.

Does it work?
Researchers have found it does seem to reduce pain in some conditions, including back pain, osteoarthritis, and ankle sprains. However, comfrey can also contain toxic substances called pyrrolizidine alkaloids that cause liver damage, cancer, and death. You should never ingest comfrey by mouth.

Is it safe?
The FDA has recommended that all oral comfrey products be removed from the market. When applied to the skin: When applied to unbroken skin in small amounts for less than 10 days, comfrey is POSSIBLY SAFE for most people. It's important to remember that the poisonous chemicals in comfrey can pass through the skin.

Cordyceps Sinensis
Sinensis is an annual Ascomycetes fungus closely related to the mushroom. Although not actually a mushroom taxonomically, it has been described as an exotic medicinal mushroom in traditional Chinese and Tibetan medicine. The name cordyceps comes from Latin words meaning club and head.

Does it work?
Cordyceps might improve immunity by stimulating cells and specific chemicals in the immune system. It might also help fight cancer cells and shrink tumor size, particularly with lung or skin cancers. Natural cordyceps is hard to get and might be expensive.

Is it safe?
Cordyceps is generally safe, but it may cause upset stomach, nausea, and dry mouth in some people. Risks. Don't take cordyceps if you have cancer, diabetes, or a bleeding disorder. Women who are pregnant or breastfeeding and children should avoid cordyceps.

Creatine
Creatine is an organic compound with the nominal formula $CNCH_2CO_2H$. It exists in various modifications in solution.

Creatine is found in vertebrates where it facilitates recycling of adenosine triphosphate, primarily in muscle and brain tissue.

Does it work?

The bottom line. At the end of the day, creatine is an effective supplement with powerful benefits for both athletic performance and health. It may boost brain function, fight certain neurological diseases, improve exercise performance, and accelerate muscle growth.

Is it safe?

Creatine is possibly safe when taken long-term. Doses up to 10 grams daily for up to 5 years have been safely used. Side effects might include dehydration, upset stomach, and muscle cramps.

Vitamin C

Vitamin C is a water-soluble vitamin found in citrus and other fruits and vegetables, and also sold as a dietary supplement. It is used to prevent and treat scurvy. Vitamin C is an essential nutrient involved in the repair of tissue, the formation of collagen, and the enzymatic production of certain neurotransmitters.

Does it work?

Vitamin C is one of the safest and most effective nutrients, experts say. Though it may not be the cure for the common cold, the benefits of vitamin C may include protection against immune system deficiencies, cardiovascular disease, prenatal health problems, eye disease, and even skin wrinkling.

Is it safe?

When taken at appropriate doses, oral vitamin C supplements are generally considered safe. Taking too much vitamin C can cause side effects, including: Nausea, vomiting and diarrhea. Heartburn.

<u>D</u>

Dandelion

Taraxacum is a large genus of flowering plants in the family Asteraceae, which consists of species commonly known as dandelions. The scientific and hobby study of the genus is known as taraxacology.

Does it work?
What's more, dandelion greens provide a substantial amount of several minerals, including iron, calcium, magnesium, and potassium .The root of the dandelion is rich in the carbohydrate inulin, a type of soluble fiber found in plants that supports the growth and maintenance of healthy gut bacteria in your digestive tract

Is it safe?
When taken by mouth: Dandelion is likely safe for most people when consumed in the amounts commonly found in food. It is possibly safe when taken in larger amounts. Dandelion might cause allergic reactions, stomach discomfort, diarrhea, or heartburn in some people.

Epigallocatechin Gallate (EGCG)
Epigallocatechin gallate, also known as epigallocatechin-3-gallate, is the ester of epigallocatechin and gallic acid, and is a type of catechin. EGCG the most abundant catechin in tea is a polyphenol under basic research for its potential to affect human health and disease.

Does it work?
Early research suggests that EGCG in green tea may play a role in improving neurological cell function and preventing degenerative brain diseases. In some studies, EGCG injections significantly improved inflammation, as well as recovery and regeneration of neural cells in mice with spinal cord injuries.

Is it safe?
It's important to note that EGCG is not 100% safe or risk-free. In fact, EGCG supplements have been associated with serious side effects, such as: liver and kidney failure.

Deer Velvet
Deer velvet covers the growing bone and cartilage that becomes deer antlers. It's sometimes used as medicine in Western countries.

Does it work?

It has no major side-effects, but based on the results of two RCTs, there's no evidence to suggest that antler velvet is effective in treating rheumatoid arthritis. Antler velvet is made from deer or elk antlers in early stages of their growth (during the velvet stage).

Is it safe?
Antler velvet may not be safe in people who should avoid supplemental estrogen, progesterone, or testosterone. The supplement may contain these hormones. Pregnant and breastfeeding women should avoid using this supplement.

Dimethyl Sulfoxide (DMSO)
Dimethyl sulfoxide is an organosulfur compound with the formula $(CH_3)_2SO$. This colorless liquid is an important polar aprotic solvent that dissolves both polar and nonpolar compounds and is miscible in a wide range of organic solvents as well as water. It has a relatively high boiling point.

Does it work?
A recent analysis of studies on the use of DMSO to relieve osteoarthritis pain found that it was not significantly more effective than placebo in relieving joint pain. There are no studies that provide guidelines for determining the proper dose of DMSO.

Is it safe?
DMSO is likely safe when used as a prescription medication. Don't use products that are not prescribed by your health professional. There is concern that some non-prescription DMSO products might be "industrial grade", which is not intended for human use.

Dehydroepiandrosterone (DHEA) (see Exercise and Athletic Performance)
Dehydroepiandrosterone, also known as androstenolone, is an endogenous steroid hormone precursor. It is one of the most abundant circulating steroids in humans. DHEA is produced in the adrenal glands, the gonads, and the brain.

Does it work?
In a small, six-week study, researchers from the National Institute of Mental Health found that treatment with DHEA

supplements helped relieve mild to moderate depression that occurs in some middle-aged people. DHEA may also be effective for improving aging skin in the elderly.

Is it safe?

DHEA is a hormone. Use of this supplement might increase levels of androgen and have a steroid effect. DHEA also might increase the risk of hormone-sensitive cancers, including prostate, breast and ovarian cancers. If you have any form of cancer or are at risk of cancer, don't use DHEA.

Devil's Claw

Native to southern Africa, devil's claw (Harpagophytum procumbens) gets its name from the tiny hooks that cover its fruit. Historically, devil's claw has been used to treat pain, liver and kidney problems, fever, and malaria. It has also been used in ointments to heal sores, boils, and other skin problems.

Does it work?

Several studies show that taking devil's claw for 8 to 12 weeks can reduce pain and improve physical functioning in people with osteoarthritis. One 4-month study of 122 people with knee and hip osteoarthritis compared devil's claw and a leading European medication for pain relief.

Is it safe?

When taken by mouth: Devil's claw is possibly safe for most adults when taken for up 12 weeks. The most common side effects are diarrhea and indigestion. Devil's claw may also cause allergic skin reactions.

Capsicum Extract Gel

This medication is used to treat minor aches and pains of the muscles/joints (such as arthritis, backache, sprains). Capsaicin works by decreasing a certain natural substance in your body (substance P) that helps pass pain signals to the brain.

Does it work?

Data from the trials was analysed together to get a single estimate of effectiveness. It was found that capsaicin was four times more effective in improving pain and joint tenderness in participants with osteoarthritis as compared to placebo gel.

Is it safe?

There are no major safety concerns in applying capsaicin gel/cream. You may feel a burning sensation when the gel touches your skin. This is because capsaicin also binds to specific receptors in nerve endings called VR1, producing a burning sensation which isn't caused by any tissue damage.

DHEA

are used by some people who believe they can improve sex drive, build muscle, fight the effects of aging, and improve some health conditions. But there isn't much evidence for many of these claims. And the supplements have some risks.Here's a rundown of what science actually knows about DHEA supplements and what you need to know about their safety.

Does it work?

A small study suggested that taking DHEA supplements might improve skin hydration and firmness, and decrease aging spots in elderly adults. Depression. DHEA might be more effective at treating depression than placebo, especially in people with low DHEA levels

Is it safe?

is a hormone. Use of this supplement might increase levels of androgen and have a steroid effect. DHEA also might increase the risk of hormone-sensitive cancers, including prostate, breast and ovarian cancers. If you have any form of cancer or are at risk of cancer, don't use

Diabetes

Diabetes is a chronic (long-lasting) health condition that affects how your body turns food into energy. Most of the food you eat is broken down into sugar (also called glucose) and released into your bloodstream. When your blood sugar goes up, it signals your pancreas to release insulin

Diatomaceous Earth

is a naturally occurring, soft, that can be crumbled into a fine powder. It has a ranging from more than 3 to less than 1 mm, but typically 10 to 200 μm. Depending on , this powder can have an feel, similar to powder, and has a low as a result of its high

Does it work?

Diatomaceous earth causes insects to dry out and die by absorbing the oils and fats from the cuticle of the insect's exoskeleton. Its sharp edges are abrasive, speeding up the process. It remains effective as long as it is kept dry and undisturbed.

Is it safe?

The Food & Drug Administration lists diatomaceous earth as generally recognized as safe. Food grade diatomaceous earth products are purified. They may be used as anticaking materials in feed, or as clarifiers for wine and beer. Always follow label instructions and take steps to minimize exposure.

Diet pills (see Weight Loss)

are tablets taken as part of a healthy diet and exercise regime to encourage weight loss. There are many kinds available, but most aren't considered effective by the NHS.Some types of diet pill may be ineffective in reducing weight. Others may be effective but considered too risky to use by UK or European medical agencies.

Does it work?

FDA-approved weight-loss diet pills aren't a magic bullet for weight loss. They won't
work for everyone, all of them have side effects, and none of them are risk-free. But the modest benefits they provide may outweigh the risks if your obesity-related health risks are significant.

Is it safe?

They can have serious effects on health. The Food and Drug Administration says many diet pills are not even legal, even ones you can find on store shelves. Many diet pill products can be tainted, contaminated or contact stimulates, which can cause major health problems or death.

Dong Quai

Dong quai (Angelica sinensis) is a plant that has been used for a variety of conditions, with little evidence. It may be unsafe when too much is consumed.Dong quai is a member of the same plant family as parsley, celery, and carrots. It's popular in Chinese medicine for female health concerns. The root might affect estrogen and other hormones.

Does it work?
Few studies have investigated dong quai for use in humans. Some lab tests suggest that dong quai contains compounds that may help reduce pain, open blood vessels, and stimulate and relax the muscles of the uterus. More studies are needed to see whether dong quai works and is safe

Is it safe?
When taken by mouth: Dong quai is possibly safe when taken for up to 6 months. It's been safely used in combination with other ingredients in doses up to 150 mg daily. It might make the skin extra sensitive to sunlight. Common side effects include burping, gas, and high blood pressure.

Vitamin D
Vitamin D (also referred to as "calciferol") is a fat-soluble vitamin that is naturally present in a few foods, added to others, and available as a dietary supplement. It is also produced endogenously when ultraviolet (UV) rays from sunlight strike the skin and trigger vitamin D synthesis.

Does it work?
How it works. Vitamin D's best-known role is to keep bones healthy by increasing the intestinal absorption of calcium. Without enough vitamin D, the body can only absorb 10% to 15% of dietary calcium, but 30% to 40% absorption is the rule when vitamin reserves are normal.

Is it safe?
Taken in appropriate doses, vitamin D is generally considered safe. However, taking too much vitamin D in the form of supplements can be harmful. Children age 9 years and older, adults, and pregnant and breastfeeding women who take more than 4,000 IU a day of vitamin D might experience: Nausea and vomiting.

E

Echinacea

Echinacea is a genus of herbaceous flowering plants in the daisy family. It has ten species, which are commonly called coneflowers. They are found only in eastern and central North America, where they grow in moist to dry prairies and open wooded area

Does it work?
Some research suggests that echinacea supplements may shorten the duration of a cold and may slightly reduce symptom severity. But these results were too minor to be considered important. Some studies have found echinacea to be helpful while other studies have found no benefit in treating colds.

Is it safe?
Echinacea is generally safe, but not for everyone. Do not take echinacea if you have any of the following conditions: an autoimmune disorder (such as lupus) multiple sclerosis

Eurycoma Longifolia
Eurycoma longifolia is a flowering plant in the family Simaroubaceae. It is native to Indochina and Indonesia, but has also been found in the Philippines. The plant is a medium-sized slender shrub that can reach 10 m in height, and is often unbranched.

Does it work?
Eurycoma longifolia is used for erectile dysfunction (ED), male infertility, increasing sexual desire in healthy people, and boosting athletic performance, but there's no good scientific evidence to support most of these uses.

Is it safe?
When taken by mouth: Eurycoma longifolia is possibly safe when taken in doses of 200 mg daily for up to 9 months or 400 mg daily for 3 months. It is possibly unsafe to use larger amounts. Some Eurycoma longifolia supplements have been found to contain mercury or lead.

Elderberry
Elderberry is one of the most commonly used medicinal plants in the world. Traditionally, Indigenous people used it to treat fever and rheumatism, while the ancient Egyptians used

it to improve their complexions and heal burns. It's still gathered and used in folk medicine across many parts of Europe.

Does it work?

The berries and flowers of elderberry are packed with antioxidants and vitamins that may boost your immune system. They could help tame inflammation, lessen stress, and help protect your heart, too. Some experts recommend elderberry to help prevent and ease cold and flu symptoms.

Is it safe?

Opinions vary on whether elderberry is helpful, but most doctors believe it's safe to have in small doses. But unripe or uncooked berries or flowers from the plant can cause nausea, vomiting, and diarrhea. Larger amounts can cause even more serious poisoning.

Eleuthero

Eleuthero (Eleutherococcus senticosus) is a woody shrub sometimes called Siberian ginseng. It is not a true ginseng. It is sometimes used as an adaptogen.

Does it work?

People use eleuthero for genital herpes, diabetes, athletic performance, memory and thinking skills, the common cold, and many other conditions, but there is no good scientific evidence to support most of these uses.

Is it safe?

Although eleuthero is likely safe when used in the short term, it may trigger a number of side effects including insomnia, headache, nervousness, upset GI tract, and diarrhea

Energy Drinks

Energy drinks are beverages that contain ingredients marketed to increase energy and mental performance. Red Bull, 5-Hour Energy, Monster, AMP, Rockstar, NOS and Full Throttle are examples of popular energy drink products.

Does it work?

In several studies, energy drinks have been found to improve physical endurance, but there's less evidence of any effect on muscle strength or power. Energy drinks may enhance alertness and improve reaction time, but they may also reduce steadiness of the hands.

Is it safe?
The American Beverage Association says "caffeine is caffeine," and where you get it from doesn't really matter. This industry group says that energy drinks are safe if you drink them in moderation.

Ephedra
Ephedra is a stimulant herb usually from the stem and branches of Ephedra sinica. Most ephedra species contain the chemical ephedrine. It's banned in the US. The ephedrine in ephedra is responsible for its therapeutic effects and also its serious safety concerns. It stimulates the heart, lungs, and nervous system.

Does it work?
Ephedra and ephedrine promote modest shortterm weight loss; their long-term effect is unknown. Ephedrine plus caffeine boosts immediate physical performance for fit young men; there is no evidence that ephedra or ephedrine improves long-term physical performance of athletes or would work for the general public.

Is it safe?
When taken by mouth: Ephedra is likely unsafe. Ephedra can cause severe side effects, such as high blood pressure, heart attacks, seizures, strokes, irregular heartbeat, and death. Taking ephedra with other stimulants like caffeine increases the risk of severe side effects.

Essiac/Flor-Essence
Essiac and Flor Essence are herbal tea mixtures that have been used as anticancer treatments. They have been used to treat other health conditions also, including diabetes, AIDS, and gastrointestinal diseases

Does it work?
There is no evidence reported in peer-reviewed scientific journals to show that the exact formulas of Essiac and Flor Essence are effective in patients with cancer or other health

conditions, or that conventional therapies interfere with the effects of Essiac.

Is it safe?

The only reported side effects caused by Essiac are nausea and vomiting. According to the company making Flor Essence, side effects may include increased bowel movements, frequent urination, swollen glands, skin blemishes, flu-like symptoms, and slight headaches

Eucalyptus

Eucalyptus is a genus of over seven hundred species of flowering trees, shrubs or mallees in the myrtle family, Myrtaceae. Along with several other genera in the tribe Eucalypteae, including Corymbia, they are commonly known as eucalypts

Does it work?

Eucalyptus leaves have many impressive benefits. They may help decrease pain, promote relaxation, and relieve cold symptoms. Many over-the-counter products also use eucalyptus extract to freshen your breath, soothe irritated skin, and repel insects.

Is it safe?

Eucalyptus contains eucalyptol, also called cineole, an organic compound that is toxic in high doses. Eucalyptus leaves are not safe for humans to eat, although eucalyptus tea contains a safe amount of eucalyptus oil.

Evening Primrose Oil

Oenothera biennis, the common evening-primrose, is a species of flowering plant in the family Onagraceae, native to eastern and central North America, from Newfoundland west to Alberta, southeast to Florida, and southwest to Texas, and widely naturalized elsewhere in temperate and subtropical regions.

Does it work?

According to an American Family Physician, evening primrose oil may help the cervix soften and efface (thin out). Other studies suggest that it can help shorten labor duration.

This is due to linolenic acid found in EPO, which may trigger a prostaglandin response in the body.

Is it safe?
Evening primrose oil is probably safe for most adults. Less is known about its safety for children. Evening primrose oil may be safe for use during pregnancy and while breastfeeding, but the evidence is not conclusive. Evening primrose oil is generally well tolerated.

Exercise and Athletic Performance
Athletic performance is an expression that is distinct from many of the broader sports science concepts, such as health, fitness, or longevity. Athletic performance describes the efforts made by an athlete to attain specific performance objectives over a period of time..Exercise involves engaging in physical activity and increasing the heart rate beyond resting levels. It is an important part of preserving physical and mental health.

Does it work?
In terms of physical effects of training, regular exercise increases muscle tone, facilitates good circulation, improves strength, agility and flexibility and improves the rate of waste product disposal.

Is it safe?
Numerous studies have been conducted to evaluate the safety and playability of traditional (non-infill) synthetic turf surfaces. Three methodologies are used to compare the safety and performance of various surfaces.

Gamma-Linolenic Acid (GLA)
gamma-Linolenic acid or GLA is a fatty acid found primarily in seed oils. When acting on GLA, arachidonate 5-lipoxygenase produces no leukotrienes and the conversion by the enzyme of arachidonic acid to leukotrienes is inhibited.

Does it work?
Taking gamma linolenic acid by mouth for 6-12 months seems to reduce symptoms and prevent nerve damage in people with nerve pain due to type 1 or type 2 diabetes. Gamma linolenic acid seems to work better in people with good blood sugar control.

Is it safe?
Gamma linolenic acid is POSSIBLY SAFE for most adults when taken by mouth in amounts of no more than 2.8 grams per day for up to a year. It can cause digestive-tract side effects, such as soft stools, diarrhea, belching, and intestinal gas. It can also make blood take longer to clot.

Vitamin E
Vitamin E is a fat-soluble vitamin with several forms, but alpha-tocopherol is the only one used by the human body. Its main role is to act as an antioxidant, scavenging loose electrons—so-called "free radicals"—that can damage cells. [1] It also enhances immune function and prevents clots from forming in heart arteries.

Does it work?
Most people get enough vitamin E from a balanced diet. If you've been diagnosed with mild to moderate Alzheimer's disease, some research suggests that vitamin E therapy might help slow disease progression. However, oral use of vitamin E might increase the risk of prostate cancer.

Is it safe?
Safety and side effects. When taken at appropriate doses, oral use of vitamin E is generally considered safe. Rarely, oral use of vitamin E can cause: Nausea

F

Fenugreek
Fenugreek is an annual plant in the family Fabaceae, with leaves consisting of three small obovate to oblong leaflets. It is cultivated worldwide as a semiarid crop. Its seeds and leaves are common ingredients in dishes from the Indian subcontinent, and have been used as a culinary ingredient since ancient times

Does it work?
Fenugreek, a type of seed, can help increase your breast milk supply. When a woman is breastfeeding, her milk supply sometimes might decrease due to stress, fatigue, or a variety of other factors. If you feel like your supply is dwindling,

consuming fenugreek can be a simple, effective way to boost your production.

Is it safe?

Fenugreek is believed to be safe in the amounts commonly found in foods. Its safety in larger doses is uncertain. It should not be used by children as a supplement. Potential side effects of fenugreek include diarrhea, nausea, and other digestive tract symptoms and rarely, dizziness and headaches.

Folinic Acid

Folinic acid, also known as leucovorin, is a medication used to decrease the toxic effects of methotrexate and pyrimethamine. It is also used in combination with 5-fluorouracil to treat colorectal cancer and pancreatic cancer, may be used to treat folate deficiency that results in anemia, and methanol poisoning.

Does it work?

In combination with fluoruracil to treat cancers such as; colon and rectal, head and neck, esophageal, and other cancers of the gastrointestinal tract. As an antidote to effects of certain chemotherapy drugs such as methotrexate. Treatment of megaloblastic anemia when folic acid deficiency is present.

Is it safe?

The side effects with treatment of leucovorin are likely attributable to other chemotherapy medications being given in combination with leucovorin. When given in combination with fluorouracil (5-FU) the side effects of fluorouracil may be more severe (see fluorocuracil). When given in combination with methotrexate, leucovorin is given to lessen the side effects of methotrexate. (see methotrexate)

Flaxseed Oil

Linseed oil, also known as flaxseed oil or flax oil, is a colourless to yellowish oil obtained from the dried, ripened seeds of the flax plant. The oil is obtained by pressing, sometimes followed by solvent extraction. Linseed oil is a drying oil, meaning it can polymerize into a solid form.

Does it work?

Flaxseed oil is high in omega-3 fatty acids and has been shown to have several health benefits, such as reduced blood pressure and improved regularity. What's more, flaxseed oil can be used in a variety of ways. It can be used as a replacement for other types of oils, added to foods or applied to your skin and hair.

Is it safe?
When taken by mouth: Flaxseed oil is likely safe for most adults. Supplements containing 2 grams of flaxseed oil daily have been used safely for up to 6 months. Higher doses of up to 24 grams daily have also been used safely for up to 7 weeks. These larger doses can cause side effects such as loose stools and diarrhea.

Feverfew
Feverfew (Tanacetum parthenium) is a flowering plant of the Asteraceae family. Its name comes from the Latin word febrifugia, meaning "fever reducer." Traditionally, feverfew was used to treat fevers and other inflammatory conditions. In fact, some people call it the "medieval aspirin"

Does it work?
Experts say that parthenolide and other ingredients in feverfew get in the way of serotonin and prostaglandin. These are natural substances that dilate the blood vessels. They may be responsible for triggering migraines. Feverfew is likely to work for migraines if taken daily for at least several months.

Is it safe?
No serious side effects have been reported from feverfew use. Side effects can include nausea, digestive problems, and bloating; if the fresh leaves are chewed, sores and irritation of the mouth may occur.

Fish Oil (see Omega-3 fatty acids)
Omega-3 fish oil contains both docosahexaenoic acid (DHA) and eicosapentaenoic acid (EPA). Omega-3 fatty acids are essential nutrients that are important in preventing and managing heart disease. Findings show omega-3 fatty acids may help to: Lower blood pressure.

Does it work?

Fish oil can lower elevated triglyceride levels. Having high levels of this blood fat puts you at risk for heart disease and stroke. Rheumatoid arthritis. Fish oil supplements (EPA+DHA) may curb stiffness and joint pain.

Is it safe?
Omega-3 fatty acids are essential for good health. Try to get them from your diet by eating fish — broiled or baked, not fried. Fish oil supplements might be helpful if you have high triglycerides or rheumatoid arthritis.

Fisetin
Fisetin is a plant flavonol from the flavonoid group of polyphenols. It can be found in many plants, where it serves as a yellow/ochre colouring agent. It is also found in many fruits and vegetables, such as strawberries, apples, persimmons, onions and cucumbers.

Does it work?
Fisetin has been shown to be an effective senolytic agent in wild-type mice, with effects of increased lifespan, reduced senescence markers in tissues, and reduced age-related pathologies.

Is it safe?
Safety: There is no evidence that fisetin would cause side effects, but no studies in humans have been conducted. There is no safety data for fisetin supplementation in humans, though no toxicity in animals has been reported.

Flaxseed
Flax (Linum usitatissimum) is a food and fiber crop. Flaxseeds are a good source of dietary fiber and omega-3 fatty acids, including alpha-linolenic acid. Flaxseeds also contain phytoestrogens called lignans, which are similar to the hormone estrogen. The fiber in flaxseed is found in the seed coat.

Does it work?
Flaxseed gel helps clumps come together easier than other styling products, and this in turn, greatly reduces frizz." The vitamin E present in flaxseed plays a significant role in fending

off damage. It's known to combat free radicals and reduce scalp inflammation.

Is it safe?

Skin sensitivity to topical gels can cause redness. Flaxseed allergy can trigger an itching reaction on the scalp and skin. Left residues of flaxseed gel can make your hair sticky and rough. Allergies to flaxseed can also cause rashes and acne

Fluoride

Fluoride is an inorganic, monatomic anion of fluorine, with the chemical formula F^-, whose salts are typically white or colorless. Fluoride salts typically have distinctive bitter tastes, and are odorless.

Does it work?

Fluoride helps because, when teeth are growing, it mixes with tooth enamel — that hard coating on your teeth. That prevents tooth decay, or cavities. But fluoride can help even after your teeth are formed. It works with saliva to protect tooth enamel from plaque and sugars.

Is it safe?

Fluoride is good for teeth, and to have good health, you need healthy teeth. Fluoride is a mineral known to be safe and effective at preventing tooth decay. There is no scientifically valid evidence to show that fluoride causes cancer, kidney disease, or other disorders.

Folate

Folate is the natural form of vitamin B9, water-soluble and naturally found in many foods. It is also added to foods and sold as a supplement in the form of folic acid; this form is actually better absorbed than that from food sources 85% vs. 50%, respectively.

Does it work?

Folic acid helps make healthy red blood cells, which carry oxygen around the body. If we do not have enough folic acid, the body can make abnormally large red blood cells that do not work properly. This causes folate deficiency anaemia, which can cause tiredness and other symptoms.

Is it safe?

Folic acid supplements are used to reduce the risk of birth defects and prevent or treat folate deficiency. They're generally considered safe if taken in recommended amounts but may interact with some prescription drugs.

Folic Acid (see Folate)
Folic acid helps make healthy red blood cells, which carry oxygen around the body. If we do not have enough folic acid, the body can make abnormally large red blood cells that do not work properly. This causes folate deficiency anaemia, which can cause tiredness and other symptoms.

Does it work?
Folic acid helps make healthy red blood cells, which carry oxygen around the body. If we do not have enough folic acid, the body can make abnormally large red blood cells that do not work properly. This causes folate deficiency anaemia, which can cause tiredness and other symptoms.

Is it safe?
When taken by mouth: It is likely safe for most people to take folic acid in doses of no more than 1 mg daily. Doses higher than 1 mg daily may be unsafe. These doses might cause stomach upset, nausea, diarrhea, irritability, confusion, behavior changes, skin reactions, seizures, and other side effects.

Forskolin (Coleus Forskohlii) (see Weight Loss)
Forskolin is made from the root of a plant in the mint family. The plant grows in Nepal, India, and Thailand. It has long been used in traditional Ayurvedic medicine.

Does it work?
Some research suggests that forskolin may aid in weight loss and muscle building. In one very small study, overweight and obese men took 250 milligrams of a 10% forskolin extract twice a day.

Is it safe?
It is not known whether taking forskolin is safe, because it has not been thoroughly studied. Some negative reactions to forskolin have been reported. These include: Flushing, fast heart beats, and low blood pressure when taken through an IV.

Fern Extract

Fern extract (Polypodiopsida or Polypodiophyta) is a member of a group of vascular plants (plants with xylem and phloem) that reproduce via spores and have neither seeds nor flowers.

Does it work?

Polypodium leucotomos is a fern from Central America. The underground runners (rhizomes) are used for medicine. Polypodium leucotomos is used to prevent certain skin problems including sunburn, eczema (atopic dermatitis), psoriasis, vitiligo, and skin cancer.

Is it safe?

Polypodium leucotomos is possibly safe when taken by mouth or applied to the skin, short-term. One polypodium leucotomos extract (Fernblock, Cantabria Farmaceutica) has been used safely for up to 2 days. Another extract (Anapsos, ASAC Pharma) has been used safely for up to 5 months.

Fucoxanthin (see Weight Loss)

Fucoxanthin comes from brown seaweed and other algae. It's claimed to help with weight loss by burning calories and decreasing fat.

Does it work?

Fucoxanthin hasn't been studied enough to know if it will help you lose weight. Only one study in people included fucoxanthin (the other studies were in animals).

Is it safe?

Fucoxanthin seems to be safe (at 2.4 mg a day for 16 weeks), but it hasn't been studied enough to know for sure.

G

Garcinia cambogia

Garcinia cambogia is a tree that grows throughout Asia, Africa, and the Polynesian islands. Hydroxycitric acid in the fruit is claimed to decrease the number of new fat cells your body makes, suppress your appetite and thus reduce the amount of food you eat, and limit the amount of weight you gain.

Does it work?
Garcinia cambogia has little to no effect on weight loss.

Is it safe?
Garcinia cambogia seems to be fairly safe. But it can cause headache, nausea, and symptoms in the upper respiratory tract, stomach, and intestines.

Garlic
Garlic (Allium sativum) is an herb related to onion, leeks, and chives. It is commonly used for conditions related to the heart and blood system. Garlic produces a chemical called allicin. This is what seems to make garlic work for certain conditions. Allicin also makes garlic smell.

Does it work?
Garlic contains antioxidants that support the body's protective mechanisms against oxidative damage. High doses of garlic supplements have been shown to increase antioxidant enzymes in humans, as well as significantly reduce oxidative stress in those with high blood pressure.

Is it safe?
When taken by mouth: Garlic is likely safe for most people. Garlic has been used safely for up to 7 years. It can cause side effects such as bad breath, heartburn, gas, and diarrhea. These side effects are often worse with raw garlic.

Gelatin
Gelatin or gelatine is a translucent, colorless, flavorless food ingredient, commonly derived from collagen taken from animal body parts. It is brittle when dry and rubbery when moist.

Does it work?
Taking gelatin might increase the production of collagen in the body. People use gelatin for aging skin, osteoarthritis, osteoporosis, brittle nails, obesity, diarrhea, and many other conditions, but there is no good scientific evidence to support these uses.

Is it safe?
When eaten in foods, gelatin is considered safe by the FDA. We don't know how safe it is to take high doses of gelatin

supplements. Some experts worry that gelatin has a risk of being contaminated with certain animal diseases. So far there have been no reported cases of people getting sick in this way.

Ginger
Ginger is a flowering plant whose rhizome, ginger root or ginger, is widely used as a spice and a folk medicine. It is a herbaceous perennial which grows annual pseudostems about one meter tall bearing narrow leaf blades

Does it work?
It's used as a food flavoring and medicine. Ginger contains chemicals that might reduce nausea and swelling. These chemicals seem to work in the stomach and intestines, but they might also help the brain and nervous system to control nausea. People commonly use ginger for many types of nausea and vomiting.

Is it safe?
When taken by mouth: Ginger is likely safe. It can cause mild side effects including heartburn, diarrhea, burping, and general stomach discomfort. Taking higher doses of 5 grams daily increases the risk for side effects. When applied to the skin: Ginger is possibly safe when used short-term.

Green-Lipped Mussel
Green-lipped mussel is a nutritional supplement taken from a type of mussel native to New Zealand. We don't really understand how it works, but it contains omega-3 fatty acids, which have anti-inflammatory and joint-protecting properties. Evidence suggests that it might be of some use to people with osteoarthritis when taken along with paracetamol or non-steroidal anti-inflammatory drugs (NSAIDs). It's not effective in treating rheumatoid arthritis.

Does it work?
Green-lipped mussel was more effective than a placebo in reducing pain, improving function and improving overall quality of life when taken along with usual painkillers (for example paracetamol) and NSAIDs.

Is it safe?

When taken by mouth: New Zealand green-lipped mussel is POSSIBLY SAFE for most people. It can cause some side effects such as itching, gout, abdominal pain, heart burn, diarrhea, nausea, and intestinal gas. In rare cases, it might cause liver problems.

Ginkgo

Ginkgo (Ginkgo biloba) is a large tree with fan-shaped leaves. The leaves are commonly included in supplements and taken by mouth for memory problems. The ginkgo tree is thought to be one of the oldest living trees, dating back more than 200 million years.

Does it work?

Ginkgo's effect on memory enhancement has had conflicting results. While some evidence suggests that ginkgo extract might modestly improve memory in healthy adults, most studies indicate that ginkgo doesn't improve memory, attention or brain function.

Is it safe?

What Do We Know About Safety? For most people, ginkgo leaf extract appears to be safe when taken by mouth in moderate amounts. Side effects of ginkgo may include headache, stomach upset, dizziness, palpitations, constipation, and allergic skin reactions.

Ginseng

Ginseng is the root of plants in the genus Panax, such as Korean ginseng, South China ginseng, and American ginseng, typically characterized by the presence of ginsenosides and gintonin.

Does it work?

It is commonly touted for its antioxidant and anti-inflammatory effects. It could also help regulate blood sugar levels and have benefits for some cancers. What's more, ginseng may strengthen the immune system, enhance brain function, fight fatigue and improve symptoms of erectile dysfunction

Is it safe?

According to research, ginseng appears to be safe and should not produce any serious adverse effects. However, people taking diabetes medications should monitor their blood sugar levels closely when using ginseng to ensure these levels do not go too low.

Glucomannan (see Weight Loss)
Glucomannan is a soluble dietary fiber from the root of the konjac plant. It's claimed to absorb water in the gut to help you feel full.

Does it work?
Glucomannan has little to no effect on weight loss. But it might help lower total cholesterol, LDL ("bad") cholesterol, triglycerides, and blood sugar levels.

Is it safe?
Most forms of glucomannan seem to be safe (at up to 15.1 g a day for several weeks in a powder or capsule form). It can cause loose stools, flatulence, diarrhea, constipation, and abdominal discomfort.

Glucosamine
Glucosamine is an amino sugar and a prominent precursor in the biochemical synthesis of glycosylated proteins and lipids. Glucosamine is part of the structure of two polysaccharides, chitosan and chitin. Glucosamine is one of the most abundant monosaccharides.

Does it work?
Some research indicates that glucosamine may reduce inflammation, especially when used alongside chondroitin supplements. Still, more research is needed on the topic.

Is it safe?
Generally safe
Glucosamine sulfate might provide some pain relief for people with osteoarthritis. The supplement appears to be safe and might be a helpful option for people who can't take nonsteroidal anti-inflammatory drugs (NSAIDs). While study results are mixed, glucosamine sulfate might be worth a try

Gingko Biloba

Ginkgo biloba, commonly known as ginkgo or gingko also known as the maidenhair tree, is a species of tree native to China. It is the last living species in the order Ginkgoales, which first appeared over 290 million years ago.

Does it work?
Ginkgo's effect on memory enhancement has had conflicting results. While some evidence suggests that ginkgo extract might modestly improve memory in healthy adults, most studies indicate that ginkgo doesn't improve memory, attention or brain function.

Is it safe?
When used orally in moderate amounts, ginkgo appears to be safe for most healthy adults. Ginkgo can cause: Headache. Dizziness.

Glutamine (see Exercise and Athletic Performance)
Glutamine is the most abundant amino acid found in the body. It's made in the muscles and transferred by the blood into different organ systems. Glutamine is a building block for making proteins in the body. It's also needed to make other amino acids and glucose.

Does it work?
Glutamine is a building block for making proteins in the body. It's also needed to make other amino acids and glucose. Glutamine supplements might help gut function, immune function, and other processes, especially in times of stress when the body uses more glutamine.

Is it safe?
Because our bodies make glutamine and it's found in many foods, it's considered safe in normal amounts. However, there are some potential health risks, so talk to your doctor before adding a glutamine supplement to your diet.

Goji
Goji, goji berry, or wolfberry, is the fruit of either Lycium barbarum or Lycium chinense, two closely related species of boxthorn in the nightshade family, Solanaceae. L. barbarum and L. chinense fruits are similar but can be distinguished by differences in taste and sugar content.

Does it work?
Antioxidants slow tumor growth, reduce inflammation, and help to remove harmful substances from the body. Research on mice, reported in the journal Drug Design, Development and Therapy, finds goji berries may inhibit tumor growth and boost the effectiveness of cancer treatments.

Is it safe?
When taken by mouth: Goji fruit is possibly safe when taken short-term. Up to 15 grams of goji fruit daily has been used safely for up to 4 months. In rare cases, goji fruit can cause allergic reactions.

Ganoderma Lucidum
Ganoderma is a genus of polypore fungi in the family Ganodermataceae that includes about 80 species, many from tropical regions. They have a high genetic diversity and are used in traditional Asian medicines. Ganoderma can be differentiated from other polypores because they have a double-walled basidiospore.

Does it work?
Reishi mushroom (Ganoderma lucidum) is a bitter-tasting fungus with no proven health benefits. It is thought to have some effects on the immune system. Reishi mushroom is used for Alzheimer disease, cancer, diabetes, cold sores, and many other conditions, but there is no good scientific evidence to support these uses.

Is it safe?
Side effects of Reishi include:Dry mouth, throat, and nose, Itchy mouth, throat, and nose, Stomach upset ,Nosebleed, Bloody stools, Rash (from reishi wine), Allergies (from breathing reishi spores)

Goldenseal
Goldenseal (Hydrastis canadensis) is an herb in the buttercup family. The dried root is very commonly used in supplements in the US. Goldenseal contains berberine, which might have effects against bacteria and fungi. Berberine also has properties that can lower blood pressure and help irregular heartbeat.

Does it work?

Goldenseal (Hydrastis canadensis) is one of the most popular herbs in the United States, often combined with echinacea and sold to treat or prevent colds. But there is no evidence that it works. In fact, there is very little scientific evidence that goldenseal works to treat any condition

Is it safe?

Goldenseal might be safe for most adults when taken by mouth in the short term. There is not enough reliable information to know if goldenseal is safe for long-term use. Women who are pregnant or breastfeeding should not use goldenseal, and it should not be given to infants.

Grape

A grape is a fruit, botanically a berry, of the deciduous woody vines of the flowering plant genus Vitis. Grapes can be eaten fresh as table grapes, used for making wine, jam, grape juice, jelly, grape seed extract, vinegar, and grape seed oil, or dried as raisins, currants and sultanas

Does it work?

The nutrients in grapes may help protect against cancer, eye problems, cardiovascular disease, and other health conditions.

Resveratrol is a key nutrient in grapes that may offer health benefits.

Grapes are a good source of fiber, potassium, and a range of vitamins and other minerals.

Grapes are suitable for people with diabetes, as long as they are accounted for in the diet plan.

Is it safe?

When taken by mouth: Grapes are commonly consumed in foods. It is possibly safe when the whole fruit or the extract of the fruit, leaf, or seed, are used as medicine. Grape seed extracts and fruit extracts have been used safely for up to 11 months. Eating large quantities of grapes might cause diarrhea.

Glycosaminoglycans

Glycosaminoglycans (GAGs), also known as mucopolysaccharides, are negatively-charged polysaccharide compounds. They are composed of repeating disaccharide units that are present in every mammalian tissue. Their functions within the body are widespread and determined by their molecular structure.

Does it work?
In conclusion, glycosaminoglycans (GAGs), have widespread functions within the body. They play a crucial role in the cell signaling process, including regulation of cell growth, proliferation, promotion of cell adhesion, anticoagulation, and wound repair.

Is it safe?
In general, glycosaminoglycan supplements are safe. However, as with any supplement, there are potential side effects and risks. Individuals who have taken glucosamine-chondroitin supplements, for example, may experience diarrhea and/or abdominal pain.

Grape Seed Extract
Grape seed extract is derived from the ground-up seeds of red wine grapes. Although fairly new to the U.S., grape seed extract is now used to treat a number of diseases.

Does it work?
There is evidence that grape seed extract is beneficial for a number of cardiovascular conditions. Grape seed extract may help with a type of poor circulation (chronic venous insufficiency) and high cholesterol. Grape seed extract also reduces swelling caused by injury and helps with eye disease related to diabetes.

Is it safe?
Grape seed extract is generally considered safe. Side effects may include headache, itchy scalp, dizziness, and nausea. Risks. People allergic to grapes should not use grape seed extract.

Grifola Frondosa
Grifola frondosa is a polypore mushroom that grows at the base of trees, particularly old growth oaks or maples. It is typically found in late summer to early autumn. It is native to China, Europe, and North America.

Does it work?
frondosa fruiting bodies or mycelial biomass have shown promising medicinal values as well. For instance, the protein components of G. frondosa, including glycoprotein, have shown anti-tumor [32], immune-enhancing [33], anti-diabetic, anti-hypertensive, anti-hyperlipidemic [34] and anti-viral effects [35].

Is it safe?
People use maitake mushroom for enlarged ovaries with cysts, diabetes, and many other conditions, but there is no good scientific evidence to support these uses.

Grapefruit
The grapefruit is a subtropical citrus tree known for its relatively large, sour to semi-sweet, somewhat bitter fruit. The interior flesh is segmented and varies in color from pale yellow to dark pink. Grapefruit is a citrus hybrid originating in Barbados.

Does it work?
Grapefruit doesn't burn fat. There have been a few studies about grapefruit and weight loss. In one, obese people who ate half a grapefruit before meals for 12 weeks lost more weight than those who didn't eat or drink any grapefruit products.

Is it safe?
Grapefruit poses a potentially lethal health risk to increasing numbers of patients taking prescription drugs, experts have warned. The fruit contains chemicals that can interact with certain drugs, making them more potent.

Gamma-Oryzanol aka Rice Bran Oil
Rice bran oil is the oil extracted from the hard outer brown layer of rice called chaff. It is known for its high smoke point of 232 °C and mild flavor, making it suitable for high-temperature cooking methods such as stir frying and deep frying.

Does it work?
Rice bran oil is also an excellent source of poly- and mono-unsaturated fats (the "good fats"). Studies have shown that consuming these unsaturated fats can improve blood

cholesterol levels, which can decrease your risk of heart disease and type 2 diabetes.

Is it safe?

Increasing the amount of bran in the diet can cause unpredictable bowel movements, intestinal gas, and stomach discomfort. Rice bran oil is considered very safe for most people when added to baths, but, it can be the reason for itching and skin redness.

Green Coffee Beans

Green coffee beans are unroasted coffee beans. Green coffee bean extract is claimed to decrease fat accumulation and help convert blood sugar into energy that your cells can use.

Does it work?

Green coffee bean extract might help you lose a small amount of weight.

Is it safe?

Green coffee bean extract seems to be safe (at up to 200 mg a day for 12 weeks). It might cause headache and urinary tract infections. Green coffee beans contain the stimulant caffeine, which can cause problems at high doses or when it's combined with other stimulants (see the section on Caffeine).

Green Tea

Green tea (also called *Camellia sinensis*) is a common beverage all over the world. Green tea and green tea extract in some weight-loss supplements are claimed to reduce body weight by increasing the calories your body burns, breaking down fat cells, and decreasing fat absorption and the amount of new fat your body makes.

Does it work?

Green tea might help you lose a small amount of weight.

Is it safe?

Drinking green tea is safe, but taking green tea extract might not be. Green tea extract can cause constipation, abdominal discomfort, nausea, and increased blood pressure. In some people, it has been linked to liver damage.

Guar Gum (see Weight Loss)

Guar gum is a soluble dietary fiber in some dietary supplements and food products. It's claimed to make you feel full, lower your appetite, and decrease the amount of food you eat.

Does it work?
Guar gum probably doesn't help you lose weight.

Is it safe?
Guar gum seems to be safe (at up to 30 g a day for 6 months) when it is taken with enough fluid. But it can cause abdominal pain, flatulence, diarrhea, nausea, and cramps.

Guarana (see Weight Loss)
Guarana (Paullinia cupana) is a plant native to the Amazon. It is a common ingredient of energy drinks and can be unsafe in large amounts. Guarana contains caffeine. Caffeine works by stimulating the central nervous system, heart, and muscles.

Does it work?
Guarana is commonly touted for its ability to reduce fatigue, boost energy and aid learning and memory. It has also been linked to better heart health, weight loss, pain relief, healthier skin, lower cancer risk and a decreased risk of age-related eye diseases.

Is it safe?
When taken by mouth: Guarana is likely safe for most adults when taken in amounts commonly found in foods. Guarana is possibly safe when taken as medicine, short-term. When taken in high doses for a long time, guarana is possibly unsafe. Guarana contains caffeine.

Glycerol
Glycerol, also called glycerine in British English and glycerin in American English, is a simple polyol compound. It is a colorless, odorless, viscous liquid that is sweet-tasting and non-toxic. The glycerol backbone is found in lipids known as glycerides.

Does it work?
People use glycerol for constipation, improving athletic performance, and for certain skin conditions. It is also used for

stroke, obesity, ear infections, and many other conditions, but there is no good scientific evidence to support these uses.

Is it safe?

When taken by mouth: Glycerol is possibly safe when used short-term. Side effects might include headaches, dizziness, bloating, nausea, and diarrhea. When applied to the skin: Glycerol is likely safe. It might cause redness, itching, and burning.

Gymnema

Gymnema is a genus in the family Apocynaceae first described as a genus in 1810. One species, Gymnema sylvestre, is commonly used as a dietary supplement and has the ability to suppress the taste of sweetness.

Does it work?

Compounds extracted from gymnema have been shown to reduce the absorption of sugar from the intestinal tract and boost insulin production, all of which could help lower blood sugar. Animal testing confirms that gymnema reduces blood glucose levels. Lab rats given gymnema extract also eat less and lose weight.

Is it safe?

Gymnema sylvestre is considered safe for most people, but it should not be taken by children or women who are pregnant, breastfeeding or planning to get pregnant. Moreover, though it appears to improve blood sugar and insulin levels, it's not a substitute for diabetes medication.

H

Hawthorn

Hawthorn is a flowering shrub in the rose family. Common species include Crataegus monogyna, Crataegus laevigata, and Crataegus oxyacantha. The hawthorn leaves, berries, and flowers are used as medicine. They contain chemicals called flavonoids, which have antioxidant effects.

Does it work?

Hawthorn can help improve the amount of blood pumped out of the heart during contractions, widen the blood vessels, and increase the transmission of nerve signals. Hawthorn also seems to have blood pressure-lowering activity, according to early research.

Is it safe?
One review of 29 clinical studies with more than 5,500 people found that hawthorn was safe when used in recommended dosages. Doses found to be safe were from 160 to 1,800 mg daily, and from 3 to 24 weeks in length. You may not notice any improvement for 6 to 12 weeks. Heart disease is a serious condition.

Hyaluronic Acid
Hyaluronic acid, also known as hyaluronan, is a clear, gooey substance that is naturally produced by your body. The largest amounts of it are found in your skin, connective tissue and eyes. Its main function is to retain water to keep your tissues well lubricated and moist.

Does it work?
There's a reason it's ubiquitous: Not only does hyaluronic acid do a killer job when it comes to moisturizing the skin, but it minimizes signs of aging, since plump, hydrated skin makes fine lines and wrinkles less visible.

Is it safe?
When taken by mouth: Hyaluronic acid is likely safe when used appropriately. Allergic reactions might occur but are rare. When applied to the skin: Hyaluronic acid is likely safe when used appropriately. Allergic reactions might occur but are rare.

Hemp
Hemp, or industrial hemp, is a botanical class of Cannabis sativa cultivars grown specifically for industrial or medicinal use. It can be used to make a wide range of products. Along with bamboo, hemp is among the fastest growing plants on Earth.

Does it work?
There's no evidence, for example, that CBD cures cancer. There is moderate evidence that CBD can improve sleep disorders, fibromyalgia pain, muscle spasticity related to

multiple sclerosis, and anxiety. People report that oral CBD helps relieve anxiety and pain and also leads to better sleep.

Is it safe?

Eating hemp seeds and hemp seed products is typically safe as part of a balanced diet. However, hemp contains antinutritional compounds that impact the absorption of minerals in the body. For example, a 2020 review found hemp seeds to be high in phytic acid, which can inhibit the absorption of iron and other minerals.

Herbal Dietary Supplements

A dietary supplement is a manufactured product intended to supplement one's diet by taking a pill, capsule, tablet, powder, or liquid. A supplement can provide nutrients either extracted from food sources or that are synthetic in order to increase the quantity of their consumption.

Does it work?

Herbal products can pose unexpected risks because many supplements contain active ingredients that have strong effects in the body.

Is it safe?

Herbal products can pose unexpected risks because many supplements contain active ingredients that have strong effects in the body. For example, taking a combination of herbal supplements or using supplements together with prescription drugs could lead to harmful, even life-threatening results.

Hibiscus

Hibiscus is a genus of flowering plants in the mallow family, Malvaceae. The genus is quite large, comprising several hundred species that are native to warm temperate, subtropical and tropical regions throughout the world.

Does it work?

The fruit acids in hibiscus may work like a laxative. Some researchers think that other chemicals in hibiscus might be able to lower blood pressure; decrease spasms in the stomach, intestines, and uterus; and work like antibiotics to kill bacteria and worms.

Is it safe?

Hibiscus sabdariffa is a plant considered safe in common food amounts. As a tea, it may be beneficial for high blood pressure.

HMB (beta-hydroxy-beta-methylbutyrate) (see Exercise and Athletic Performance)

β-Hydroxy β-methylbutyric acid (HMB), otherwise known as its conjugate base, β-hydroxy β-methylbutyrate, is a naturally produced substance in humans that is used as a dietary supplement and as an ingredient in certain medical foods that are intended to promote wound healing and provide nutritional support for people with muscle wasting due to cancer or HIV/AIDS. In healthy adults, supplementation with HMB has been shown to increase exercise-induced gains in muscle size, muscle strength, and lean body mass, reduce skeletal muscle damage from exercise, improve aerobic exercise performance, and expedite recovery from exercise.

Does it work?

HMB might promote muscle growth. It seems to reduce the destructive breakdown of muscle in people with AIDS.

Is it safe?

The leucine metabolite, beta-hydroxy-beta-methylbutyrate (HMB) enhances the effects of exercise on muscle size and strength. Although several reports in animals and humans indicate that HMB is safe, quantitative safety data in humans have not been reported definitively.

Hoodia

Hoodia is a plant from southern Africa, where it's used as an appetite suppressant.

Does it work?

There hasn't been much research on hoodia, but it probably won't help you eat less or lose weight. Analyses showed that some "hoodia" supplements sold in the past contained very little hoodia or none at all. It's not known whether this is true of hoodia supplements sold today.

Is it safe?

Hoodia might not be safe. It can cause rapid heart rate, increased blood pressure, headache, dizziness, nausea, and vomiting.

Hops

Hops are the green cone-shaped flowers, or "inflorescence," of the Humulus lupulus plant. They're a climbing perennial with a distinct jackpot for craft brewers. Hidden inside each cone are tiny yellow pods or glands called lupulin—the source of bitterness, aroma, and flavor in beer.

Does it work?

Early scientific studies found no solid evidence to support claims of hops' sleep-inducing potential. More recently, researchers have taken a closer look at hops and their effect on anxiety and sleep disorders. Several scientific studies suggest that hops do have sedative effects.

Is it safe?

Hops extracts and hops bitter acids are possibly safe when used short-term. Hops extracts have been used safely in doses of up to 300 mg daily for up to 3 months. Hops bitter acids have been used safely in doses of 35 mg daily for 3 months. Hops might cause dizziness and sleepiness in some people.

Horny Goat Weed

Epimedium, also known as barrenwort, bishop's hat, fairy wings, horny goat weed, or yin yang huo, is a genus of flowering plants in the family Berberidaceae. The majority of the species are endemic to China, with smaller numbers elsewhere in Asia, and a few in the Mediterranean region.

Does it work?

People use horny goat weed for erectile dysfunction (ED), sexual problems, weak and brittle bones, health problems after menopause, and other conditions, but there is no good scientific evidence to support any of these uses.

Is it safe?

When taken by mouth: Horny goat weed extract is possibly safe when used short-term. A specific extract of horny goat weed containing phytoestrogens has been taken by mouth safely for up to 2 years. Another extract containing a chemical called icariin has been taken safely for up to 6 months.

Horse Chestnut

Aesculus hippocastanum, the horse chestnut, is a species of flowering plant in the soapberry and lychee family Sapindaceae. It is a large deciduous, synoecious tree. It is also called horse-chestnut, European horsechestnut, buckeye, and conker tree. It is sometimes called Spanish chestnut.

Does it work?

The bottom line. Horse chestnut extract has powerful anti-inflammatory properties and may help relieve pain and inflammation caused by chronic venous insufficiency (CVI). It may also benefit other health conditions like hemorrhoids and male infertility caused by swollen veins.

Is it safe?

Raw horse chestnut seed, bark, flower, and leaf contain esculin and are unsafe to use. Signs of esculin poisoning include stomach upset, muscle twitching, weakness, vomiting, diarrhea, depression, and paralysis. Seek immediate medical attention if you've accidentally consumed raw horse chestnut.

Horsetail

Horsetail (Equisetum arvense) is an herbal remedy that dates back to ancient Roman and Greek times. It was used traditionally to stop bleeding, heal ulcers and wounds, and treat tuberculosis and kidney problems. The name Equisetum is derived from the Latin roots equus, meaning "horse," and seta, meaning "bristle."

Does it work?

They might also work like "water pills" (diuretics) and increase urination. People use horsetail for fluid retention, urinary tract infections (UTIs), osteoporosis, loss of bladder control, and many other conditions, but there is no good scientific evidence to support these uses.

Is it safe?

Horsetail remedies prepared from Equisetum arvense are generally considered safe when used properly. Another species of horsetail, however, called Equisetum palustre is poisonous to horses. To be safe, never take that form of horsetail. Be sure to buy products made by an established company with a good reputation

Huperzine A

Huperzine A is a naturally occurring sesquiterpene alkaloid compound found in the firmoss Huperzia serrata and in varying quantities in other food Huperzia species, including H. elmeri, H. carinat, and H. aqualupian.

Does it work?

Some studies have found evidence that huperzine A might significantly improve cognitive performance in people with Alzheimer's disease. However, a recent systematic review found that the quality of the evidence of huperzine A's effectiveness was low.

Is it safe?

When taken by mouth: Huperzine A is possibly safe when taken for less than 6 months. It can cause some side effects including nausea, diarrhea, vomiting, dry mouth, constipation, sweating, and blurred vision.

Hydroxycitric Acid (garcinia cambogia) (see Weight Loss)

Hydroxycitric acid (HCA) is an active ingredient extracted from the rind of the Indian fruit Garcinia cambogia. It inhibits adenosine triphosphate citrate lyase and has been used in the treatment of obesity.

Does it work?

How does it work? Hydroxycitric acid might improve weight loss by preventing fat storage and controlling appetite. It might improve exercise performance by limiting the use of stored energy in the muscles, which seems to prevent fatigue.

Is it safe?

Garcinia cambogia-derived hydroxycitric acid (HCA) is a safe, natural supplement for weight management. HCA is a competitive inhibitor of ATP citrate lyase, a key enzyme which facilitates the synthesis of fatty acids, cholesterol and triglycerides.

Hydroxytryptophan (5-HTP)

5-Hydroxytryptophan, also known as oxitriptan, is a naturally occurring amino acid and chemical precursor as well as a metabolic intermediate in the biosynthesis of the neurotransmitter serotonin.

Does it work?
It found that supplementing with 5-HTP daily for six months prevented or significantly decreased the number of migraine attacks in 71% of participants. In another study in 48 students, 5-HTP produced a 70% decrease in headache frequency, compared to an 11% decrease in the placebo group.

Is it safe?
When taken by mouth: It is possibly safe to take 5-HTP in doses of up to 400 mg daily for up to one year. The most common side effects include heartburn, stomach pain, nausea, vomiting, diarrhea, drowsiness, sexual problems, and muscle problems. Large doses of 5-HTP, such as 6-10 grams daily, are possibly unsafe.

I

Iodine
Iodine is a trace element that is naturally present in some foods, is added to some types of salt, and is available as a dietary supplement. Iodine is an essential component of the thyroid hormones thyroxine (T4) and triiodothyronine (T3).

Does it work?
Iodine is a mineral found in some foods. The body needs iodine to make thyroid hormones. These hormones control the body's metabolism and many other important functions. The body also needs thyroid hormones for proper bone and brain development during pregnancy and infancy.

Is it safe?
When taken by mouth: Iodine is likely safe for most people when taken in doses less than 1100 mcg daily. Large amounts or long-term use of iodine is possibly unsafe. Adults should avoid prolonged use of higher doses without proper medical supervision.

Inositol

Inositol, or more precisely myo-inositol, is a carbocyclic sugar that is abundant in the brain and other mammalian tissues; it mediates cell signal transduction in response to a variety of hormones, neurotransmitters, and growth factors and participates in osmoregulation.

Does it work?
Research suggests that inositol may aid people with mental health and metabolic conditions, such as panic disorder, depression, bipolar disorder, polycystic ovary syndrome, metabolic syndrome and diabetes. It appears to be safe for most people and cause only mild if any side effects in daily doses up to 18 grams.

Is it safe?
Inositol is generally considered safe in adults. Side effects, if any, tend to be mild and may include nausea, stomach pain, tiredness, headache, and dizziness. Most side effects occur with doses greater than 12 grams per day. The metabolic effects of inositol may not be appropriate for everyone.

Isoflavones
Isoflavones are substituted derivatives of isoflavone, a type of naturally occurring isoflavonoids, many of which act as phytoestrogens in mammals. Isoflavones are produced almost exclusively by the members of the bean family, Fabaceae.

Does it work?
A 2015 analysis of 10 studies found that plant isoflavones from soy and other sources reduced hot flashes by 11 percent. Although many studies show that soy and soy isoflavones can modestly reduce the number and severity of hot flashes, it doesn't seem to work as quickly as hormone replacement therapy.

Is it safe?
Unconjugated soy isoflavones appear to be safe and well tolerated in healthy postmenopausal women at doses of 900 mg per day.

Iron
Iron is a major component of hemoglobin, a type of protein in red blood cells that carries oxygen from your lungs to all

parts of the body. Without enough iron, there aren't enough red blood cells to transport oxygen, which leads to fatigue.

Does it work?
Iron helps red blood cells carry oxygen from the lungs to cells all over the body. Iron also plays a role in many important functions in the body. People commonly use iron for preventing and treating different types of anemia caused by low iron levels.

Is it safe?
Yes, iron can be harmful if you get too much. In healthy people, taking high doses of iron supplements (especially on an empty stomach) can cause an upset stomach, constipation, nausea, abdominal pain, vomiting, and fainting. High doses of iron can also decrease zinc absorption

Isoleucine (see Exercise and Athletic Performance)
Isoleucine is an essential amino acid. It may help how hemoglobin is made. This is the oxygen-carrying pigment inside of red blood cells. It may help control blood sugar. It may also boost energy and endurance.

Does it work?
Isoleucine, as one of the branched chain amino acids, is also critical in physiological functions of the whole body, such as growth, immunity, protein metabolism, fatty acid metabolism and glucose transportation. Isoleucine can improve the immune system, including immune organs, cells and reactive substances.

Is it safe?
l-Isoleucine produced using C. glutamicum KCCM 80189 is considered safe for the target species, for the consumer and for the environment. l-Isoleucine produced by C. glutamicum KCCM 80189 is considered not toxic by inhalation, not irritant to skin or eyes and not a dermal sensitiser.

Inulin
Inulin is a type of prebiotic. It's not digested or absorbed in the stomach. It stays in the bowel and helps certain beneficial bacteria to grow. Inulin is a starchy substance found in a wide

variety of fruits, vegetables, and herbs, including wheat, onions, bananas, leeks, artichokes, and asparagus.

Does it work?
People commonly use inulin by mouth for weight loss, constipation, and diabetes. It's also used for high blood fats, including cholesterol and triglycerides, and many other conditions, but there is no good scientific evidence to support most of these uses.

Is it safe?
When taken by mouth: Inulin is likely safe for most people in the amounts found in foods. It is possibly safe in adults when taken as a supplement, short-term. Doses of 8-18 grams daily have been used safely for 6-12 weeks. The most common side effects include gas, bloating, diarrhea, constipation, and cramps.

K

Kava
Kava or kava kava is a crop of the Pacific Islands. The name kava is from Tongan and Marquesan, meaning 'bitter'; other names for kava include 'awa, 'ava, yaqona or yagona, sakau, seka, and malok or malogu.

Does it work?
Studies have shown that the properties in kava can ease anxiety, relieve stress, and relax muscle and nervous tension, as well as combat insomnia and improve sleep problems. That's why many people who consume kava use it a natural alternative to anti-anxiety medication.

Is it safe?
Kava has a long history of consumption in the South Pacific and is considered a safe and enjoyable beverage. The roots of the plant contain compounds called kavalactones, which have been shown to help with anxiety. Consult your doctor if you plan on taking kava, as it may interact with some medications.

Ketones
Ketones are substances that your body makes if your cells don't get enough glucose (blood sugar). Glucose is your body's

main source of energy. Ketones can show up in blood or urine. High ketone levels may indicate diabetic ketoacidosis (DKA), a complication of diabetes that can lead to a coma or even death.

Does it work?
Ketone supplements have been shown to decrease appetite, which may help you lose weight by eating less. In one study in 15 people of normal weight, those drinking a beverage containing ketone esters experienced 50% less hunger after an overnight fast than those drinking a sugary beverage.

Is it safe?
For most people, producing small amounts of ketone bodies is perfectly safe and can even be desirable. Every living animal possesses the capability of switching from sugar to ketones for fuel.

Kola Nut (Cola Nut) (see Weight Loss)
The term kola nut usually refers to the seeds of certain species of plant of the genus Cola, placed formerly in the cocoa family Sterculiaceae and now usually subsumed in the mallow family Malvaceae. These cola species are trees native to the tropical rainforests of Africa.

Does it work?
Aid to digestion: Kola nut powder and extract may help digestion. They are thought to promote the production of gastric acid, which increases digestive enzyme effectiveness in the stomach. Increase in circulation: The caffeine and theobromine in the kola nut may speed up the heart rate, which increases circulation.

Is it safe?
Kola nut has been listed by the U.S. Food and Drug Administration (FDA) as generally safe for human consumption. Kola nut extract is classified as a natural food flavoring. The FDA has also approved kola extract as an inactive ingredient in certain pharmaceuticals.

Vitamin K
Vitamin K refers to structurally similar, fat-soluble vitamers found in foods and marketed as dietary supplements. The human body requires vitamin K for post-synthesis modification

of certain proteins that are required for blood coagulation or for controlling binding of calcium in bones and other tissues.

Does it work?

Vitamin K helps to make four of the 13 proteins needed for blood clotting, which stops wounds from continuously bleeding so they can heal. People who are prescribed anticoagulants (also called blood thinners) to prevent blood clots from forming in the heart, lung, or legs are often informed about vitamin K.

Is it safe?

When taken by mouth: The two forms of vitamin K (vitamin K1 and vitamin K2) are likely safe when taken appropriately. Vitamin K1 10 mg daily and vitamin K2 45 mg daily have been safely used for up to 2 years. It's usually well-tolerated, but some people may have an upset stomach or diarrhea.

L

L-arginine

Arginine, also known as l-arginine, is an α-amino acid that is used in the biosynthesis of proteins. It contains an α-amino group, an α-carboxylic acid group, and a side chain consisting of a 3-carbon aliphatic straight chain ending in a guanidino group.

Does it work?

Generally safe. L-arginine is considered to be generally safe. It might be effective at lowering blood pressure, reducing the symptoms of angina and PAD , and treating erectile dysfunction due to a physical cause. However, if you take a blood pressure drug, talk to your doctor before using L-arginine.

Is it safe?

L-arginine is considered to be generally safe. It might be effective at lowering blood pressure, reducing the symptoms of angina and PAD , and treating erectile dysfunction due to a physical cause.

L-Tryptophan

L-tryptophan is an essential amino acid that helps the body make proteins and certain brain-signaling chemicals. Your body changes L-tryptophan into a brain chemical called serotonin. Serotonin helps control your mood and sleep.

Does it work?

The theory is that these conditions may be linked to a problem with serotonin processing in the body, and that L-tryptophan could help that. However, there is little evidence to show this really works. Early research in people hints that L-tryptophan supplements may be helpful for: Obstructive sleep apnea.

Is it safe?

L-tryptophan supplements are possibly safe when taken for up to 3 weeks. L-tryptophan can cause some side effects such as drowsiness, stomach pain, vomiting, diarrhea, headache, blurry vision, and others. In 1989, L-tryptophan was linked to cases of a neurological condition called eosinophilia-myalgia syndrome (EMS).

Lactobacillus

Lactobacillus species are probiotics ("good" bacteria) normally found in human digestive and urinary tracts. They can be consumed for diarrhea and "gut health." "Good" bacteria such as Lactobacillus can help the body break down food, absorb nutrients, and fight off "bad" organisms that might cause diseases.

Does it work?

Lactobacillus species are probiotics ("good" bacteria) normally found in human digestive and urinary tracts. They can be consumed for diarrhea and "gut health." "Good" bacteria such as Lactobacillus can help the body break down food, absorb nutrients, and fight off "bad" organisms that might cause diseases.

Is it safe?

Lactobacillus is likely safe for adults, children, and babies. Pregnant and breastfeeding women have also used one type of lactobacillus safely. But other types of lactobacillus need more study to be sure they are safe and effective.

Lavender

Lavender (Lavandula angustifolia) is an evergreen plant native to the Mediterranean. Its flower and oil have a popular scent and are also used as medicine. Lavender contains an oil that seems to have calming effects and might relax certain muscles. It also seems to have antibacterial and antifungal effects.

Does it work?
There is growing evidence suggesting that lavender oil may be an effective medicament in treatment of several neurological disorders. Several animal and human investigations suggest anxiolytic, mood stabilizer, sedative, analgesic, and anticonvulsive and neuroprotective properties for lavender.

Is it safe?
Consumption of lavender in the amounts typically used in foods is likely to be safe. Short-term oral use in the amounts tested in studies of lavender for anxiety or other conditions may also be safe. The topical use of products containing lavender may cause allergic skin reactions in some people.

Leucine (see Exercise and Athletic Performance)
Leucine is one of the 3 essential branched chain amino acids (BCAAs). These amino acids can be used by skeletal muscle to give energy during exercise. Eating foods that have complete protein gives enough of these amino acids. This includes foods such as meat, poultry, fish, eggs, and milk.

Does it work?
Results of studies have not been reliable in showing that taking supplements of these amino acids improves exercise performance, builds muscle mass, or helps you recover from exercise. Leucine may help in healing skin and bones. It may increase muscle growth and lean body mass.

Is it safe?
Very high doses of leucine may cause low blood sugar (hypoglycemia). It may also cause pellagra. Symptoms of this can include skin lesions, hair loss, and gastrointestinal problems. People who are pregnant or breastfeeding shouldn't use leucine supplements.

Licorice Root

Liquorice or licorice is the common name of Glycyrrhiza glabra, a flowering plant of the bean family Fabaceae, from the root of which a sweet, aromatic flavouring can be extracted. The liquorice plant is an herbaceous perennial legume native to Western Asia, North Africa, and Southern Europe.

Does it work?
Licorice root may have potent antioxidant, anti-inflammatory, and antimicrobial effects. Early research suggests that, as a result, it may ease upper respiratory infections, treat ulcers, and aid digestion, among other benefits.

Is it safe?
Although licorice root is generally considered safe as a food ingredient, it can cause serious side effects, including increased blood pressure and decreased potassium levels, when consumed in large amounts or for long periods of time.

Lutein
Lutein is a type of organic pigment called a carotenoid. It is related to beta-carotene and vitamin A. Many people think of lutein as "the eye vitamin." Lutein is one of two major carotenoids found in the human eye (macula and retina).

Does it work?
Lutein is a carotenoid with reported anti-inflammatory properties. A large body of evidence shows that lutein has several beneficial effects, especially on eye health. In particular, lutein is known to improve or even prevent age-related macular disease which is the leading cause of blindness and vision impairment.

Is it safe?
When taken by mouth: Lutein is likely safe when taken by mouth. Consuming up to 20 mg of lutein daily as part of the diet or as a supplement appears to be safe.

Medicinal Mushrooms
Medicinal fungi are fungi which contain metabolites or can be induced to produce metabolites through biotechnology to develop prescription drugs.

Does it work?

There is no scientific evidence supporting the use of mushroom extracts in the treatment of disease. Claims about the miraculous properties of medicinal mushrooms should be evaluated critically. Secondary metabolites with useful pharmacological properties may be widespread in mushrooms.

Is it safe?
Medicinal mushrooms have been approved adjuncts to standard cancer treatments in Japan and China for more than 30 years and have an extensive clinical history of safe use as single agents or combined with chemotherapy. The reishi mushroom is also known as lingzhi.

Lycopene
Lycopene is a type of organic pigment called a carotenoid. It is related to beta-carotene and gives some vegetables and fruits (e.g., tomatoes) a red color. Lycopene is a powerful antioxidant that might help protect cells from damage.

Does it work?
Lycopene is a powerful antioxidant with many health benefits, including sun protection, improved heart health and a lower risk of certain types of cancer. Though it can be found as a supplement, it may be most effective when consumed from lycopene-rich foods like tomatoes and other red or pink fruits.

Is it safe?
When consumed in foods, lycopene is safe to eat for everyone. Eating excessive amounts of lycopene could lead to a condition called lycopenemia, which is an orange or red discoloration of the skin. The condition itself is harmless and goes away by eating a diet lower in lycopene.

Lutein and Zeaxanthin
Lutein and zeaxanthin are yellow carotenoid antioxidants known as macular pigments. They are concentrated in the macula, the central part of your retina, which is a layer of light-sensitive cells on the back wall of your eyeball. Lutein and zeaxanthin function as a natural sunblock.

Does it work?
Lutein and zeaxanthin can help protect your eyes from harmful high-energy light waves like ultraviolet rays in

sunlight. Studies suggest that a high level of both in eye tissue is linked with better vision, especially in dim light or where glare is a problem.

Is it safe?
Though there are very few reported side effects of lutein and zeaxanthin supplements, more research is needed to evaluate the potential side effects of very high intakes. Lutein and zeaxanthin are overall safe to supplement at the recommended doses, but skin yellowing may occur over time.

Lentinus edodes
Lentinus edodes is the first medicinal macrofungus to enter the realm of modern biotechnology. It is the second most popular edible mushroom in the global market which is attributed not only to its nutritional value but also to possible potential for therapeutic applications.

Does it work?
Lentinan might increase the effects of certain medications that fight viruses and cancer. It might also increase the activity of some of the body's defense (immune) cells.

Is it safe?
The Panel concludes that the novel food Lentinex is safe as a food ingredient at the proposed conditions of use and the proposed levels of intake. 1. Dossier on Lentinex® derived from the Mushroom Lentinus edodes received on 21 October 2009.

M

Maca
Lepidium meyenii, known as maca or Peruvian ginseng, is an edible herbaceous biennial plant of the family Brassicaceae that is native to South America in the high Andes mountains of Peru. It was found exclusively at the Meseta de Bombón plateau close to Lake Junin in the late 1980s.

Does it work?
Claims that maca is a highly effective aphrodisiac may be exaggerated, Berman says. "Some claims are over the top -- compared to a placebo, maca only slightly enhanced sexual

desire. The strongest evidence is that it may increase sperm count and improve fertility in certain men,"

Is it safe?

When taken by mouth: Maca is likely safe for most people when eaten in foods. Maca is possibly safe when taken in larger amounts as medicine, short-term. Doses up to 3 grams daily seem to be safe when taken for up to 4 months.

Magnesium

Magnesium is a cofactor in more than 300 enzyme systems that regulate diverse biochemical reactions in the body, including protein synthesis, muscle and nerve function, blood glucose control, and blood pressure regulation [1-3]. Magnesium is required for energy production, oxidative phosphorylation, and glycolysis.

Does it work?

Magnesium plays many crucial roles in the body, such as supporting muscle and nerve function and energy production. Low magnesium levels usually don't cause symptoms. However, chronically low levels can increase the risk of high blood pressure, heart disease, type 2 diabetes and osteoporosis.

Is it safe?

When taken by mouth: Magnesium is likely safe for most people when taken appropriately. Doses less than 350 mg daily are safe for most adults. In some people, magnesium might cause stomach upset, nausea, vomiting, diarrhea, and other side effects.

MCT Oil

MCT oil is a supplement made from a type of fat called medium-chain triglycerides.

Does it work?

MCT can help your body make ketones, an energy source for your brain that doesn't have carbs. Some say drinking it will make your mind sharper. But if you don't have a cognitive disorder, you aren't likely to get a long-lasting brain boost just by adding some MCT oil.

Is it safe?

It's generally safe to use MCT oil moderately. But you should be careful when using it long-term. Some of the negatives include: It has a lot of calories.

Moringa Leaf Powder
Moringa oleifera is a plant that is often called the drumstick tree, the miracle tree, the ben oil tree, or the horseradish tree.

Does it work?
Moringa powder can be used to protect tissue (liver, kidneys, heart, and lungs), and to reduce pain. Antioxidants help protect cells against free radicals, which are produced by digesting food, smoking, and exposure to radiation. Antioxidants from plant-based sources such as moringa powder are considered best.

Is it safe?
Amounts and Dosage. Consuming moringa powder is proven to be safe, even at higher levels. Daily dosage should be limited to the equivalent of 70 grams of moringa leaves per day or 11 teaspoons of moringa powder.

Marshmallow Root
Althaea is a genus of herbaceous perennial plants native to Europe, North Africa and western Asia. It includes Althaea officinalis, also known as the marshmallow plant, whence the fluffy confection got its name. They are found on the banks of rivers and in salt marshes, preferring moist, sandy soils.

Does it work?
The mucilage may have a soothing effect on the esophagus by coating it. The results of several small studies have suggested that herbal cough remedies that contain marshmallow root can have this effect. One study found that marshmallow root lozenges or syruphelped treat a dry cough.

Is it safe?
When taken by mouth: Marshmallow root and leaf are likely safe when taken in the amounts found in foods. It is possibly safe to take the root and leaf in larger amounts as medicine.

Manganese
Manganese is a chemical element with the symbol Mn and atomic number 25. It is a hard, brittle, silvery metal, often

found in minerals in combination with iron. Manganese is a transition metal with a multifaceted array of industrial alloy uses, particularly in stainless steels.

Does it work?

Manganese is a trace mineral. It is vital for the human body, but people only need it in small amounts. Manganese contributes to many bodily functions, including the metabolism of amino acids, cholesterol, glucose, and carbohydrates. It also plays a role in bone formation, blood clotting, and reducing inflammation.

Is it safe?

When taken by mouth: Manganese is likely safe for most adults when taken by mouth in amounts up to 11 mg per day. However, people who have trouble getting rid of manganese from the body, such as people with liver disease, may experience side effects when taking less than 11 mg per day.

Mangosteen

Mangosteen (Garcinia mangostana) is a plant that grows in Southeast Asia. The fruit is dark purple or red. The fruit pulp is slightly acidic and sweet. Mangosteen contains chemicals that might act as antioxidants and fight infections.

Does it work?

Recent scientific studies suggest that mangosteen possesses strong antioxidant, anti-cancer, anti-inflammatory, anti-allergic, anti-microbial, and anti-malarial properties. Xanthone and vitamins in mangosteen are considered the major active components.

Is it safe?

Very few adverse health effects have been reported from consuming mangosteen in its whole form, and it's likely safe for most people. However, more concentrated forms — like supplements, juices, or powders — are not 100% risk-free.

Maritime Pine

Pinus pinaster, the maritime pine or cluster pine, is a pine native to the Mediterranean region. It is a hard, fast growing pine containing small seeds with large wings.

Does it work?

Maritime pine contains chemicals that might improve blood flow, stimulate the immune system, reduce swelling, prevent infections, and have antioxidant effects. Maritime pine trees that grow in southwest France are used to make Pycnogenol, the trademarked name for a specific maritime pine bark extract. Maritime pine bark extract is used for asthma, high cholesterol, decline in memory, ADHD, and many other conditions, but there is no good scientific evidence to support many of these uses.

Is it safe?
When taken by mouth: A specific maritime pine bark extract (Pycnogenol) is possibly safe when taken in doses of 50-450 mg daily for up to one year. It might cause dizziness and stomach problems in some people.

Melatonin
Melatonin is a hormone primarily released by the pineal gland at night, and has long been associated with control of the sleep–wake cycle. As a dietary supplement, it is often used for the short-term treatment of insomnia, such as from jet lag or shift work, and is typically taken orally.

Does it work?
Melatonin is an effective supplement that may help you fall asleep, especially if you have insomnia or jet lag. It may offer other health benefits as well.

Is it safe?
Melatonin is generally safe for short-term use. Unlike with many sleep medications, with melatonin you are unlikely to become dependent, have a diminished response after repeated use (habituation), or experience a hangover effect. The most common melatonin side effects include: Headache.

Menopause
Menopause is a point in time 12 months after a woman's last period. The years leading up to that point, when women may have changes in their monthly cycles, hot flashes, or other symptoms, are called the menopausal transition or perimenopause. The menopausal transition most often begins between ages 45 and 55.

Does it work?
The menopause is caused by changes in hormone levels which take place as a woman gets older. Menopausal symptoms include hot flushes, mood changes, memory problems and changes in sex drive. The length of time that symptoms last for varies between individuals, but averages about 4 years.

Is it safe?
Heart and blood vessel (cardiovascular) disease. When your estrogen levels decline, your risk of cardiovascular disease increases. Osteoporosis. This condition causes bones to become brittle and weak, leading to an increased risk of fractures, urinary incontinence, sexual function, and weight gain.

Methylsulfonylmethane (MSM)
Methylsulfonylmethane (MSM) is a chemical that occurs naturally in humans, as well as some green plants and animals. It can also be made in a lab. MSM might supply sulfur to make other chemicals in the body.

Does it work?
But researchers have more work to do to confirm this. MSM has shown some effectiveness for treating allergies, repetitive stress injuries, certain bladder disorders like interstitial cystitis, and wounds, but more research is needed before it can be recommended for any of these conditions.

Is it safe?
As a Generally Recognized As Safe (GRAS) approved substance, MSM is well-tolerated by most individuals at dosages of up to four grams daily, with few known and mild side effects.

Milk Thistle
Silybum marianum has other common names including cardus marianus, milk thistle, blessed milkthistle, Marian thistle, Mary thistle, Saint Mary's thistle, Mediterranean milk thistle, variegated thistle and Scotch thistle. This species is an annual or biennial plant of the family Asteraceae.

Does it work?

Medical research on milk thistle and liver health has led to mixed results. Studies show that silymarin may help ease inflammation and promote cell repair. This may help ease symptoms from liver diseases like jaundice, cirrhosis, liver cancer, and fatty liver disease.

Is it safe?
Taken in appropriate doses, oral use of milk thistle appears to be safe. Milk thistle can cause: Gastrointestinal issues, such as diarrhea, constipation, nausea, vomiting and abdominal bloating.

Mistletoe
Mistletoes are parasitic plants of the families Loranthaceae, Misodendraceae, and Santalaceae. The many species of mistletoe are slow-growing but persistent, and they are pests of many ornamental, timber, and crop trees. Some species are used as Christmas decorations.

Does it work?
Some research suggests that mistletoe may be beneficial for improving quality of life, decreasing treatment-related side effects, increasing survival time, and improving symptoms in people with certain cancers.

Is it safe?
In reality, studies show that mistletoe is not quite as hazardous as it is made out to be. The plant does in fact contain harmful chemicals like viscotoxins, which can cause gastrointestinal distress, a slowed heartbeat and other reactions.

Mitochondrial disorders (see Primary Mitochondrial Disorders)
Mitochondrial diseases are long-term, genetic, often inherited disorders that occur when mitochondria fail to produce enough energy for the body to function properly. One in 5,000 individuals has a genetic mitochondrial disease.

Ma Huang
The 3 species of this shrubby plant that are sources of the drug are native to China, where the aboveground parts are collected in the fall and dried for drug use. The root of E. sinica

or E. intermedia is known as ma huang gen and is considered to be a distinct drug, used for its anti-soporific (anti-sleep) properties.

Does it work?

While asthma treatment is one of the classical clinical uses for pure ephedrine as a pharmaceutical drug, dietary supplements promote ephedra as the herb for weight loss and increasing athletic performance. Ephedra has been a major component of herbal supplements for weight loss and athletic performance, often with caffeine also added. However, many manufacturers have recently reformulated products to remove ephedra because of legal liability questions. Because of its potential serious side effects, its use is not recommended.

Is it safe?

Ephedra use has been linked to cardiovascular adverse effects, including hypertension, stroke, and MI. Patients with hyperthyroidism, benign prostatic hyperplasia, glaucoma, diabetes mellitus, and seizures and women who are pregnant should exercise particular caution.

Molybdenum

Molybdenum is an essential trace mineral. It is found in foods such as milk, cheese, cereal grains, legumes, nuts, leafy vegetables, and organ meats. Molybdenum is most commonly used for molybdenum deficiency.

Does it work?

What is molybdenum and what does it do? Molybdenum is a mineral that you need to stay healthy. Your body uses molybdenum to process proteins and genetic material like DNA. Molybdenum also helps break down drugs and toxic substances that enter the body.

Is it safe?

Molybdenum is safe in amounts that do not exceed 2 mg per day, the tolerable upper intake level. However, molybdenum is possibly unsafe when taken by mouth in high doses. Adults should avoid exceeding 2 mg daily.

Multivitamin/mineral Supplements

Multivitamin/mineral (MVM) supplements contain a combination of vitamins and minerals, and sometimes other ingredients as well. People refer to them by many names, including multis and multiples or simply vitamins. Each of the vitamins and minerals in MVMs have a unique role in the body. For more information about each one, see our individual vitamin and mineral fact sheets.

Does it work?

The researchers concluded that multivitamins don't reduce the risk for heart disease, cancer, cognitive decline (such as memory loss and slowed-down thinking) or an early death. They also noted that in prior studies, vitamin E and beta-carotene supplements appear to be harmful, especially at high doses.

Is it safe?

Despite a balanced and overall healthy diet, micronutrient gaps may occur from time to time. An MVM can help to improve the nutrient supply and overcome problems of inadequacy without concern for its long-term safety. MVM are safe for long-term use (more than 10 y) as documented in a recent clinical trial.

Mushrooms

Mushrooms are edible fungus that can provide several important nutrients. The many kinds of mushroom have varying compositions and nutritional profiles. From puffballs to truffles, mushrooms can range from everyday fare to a costly delicacy. People can buy them fresh, canned, or dried.

Does it work?

As an excellent source of both fiber and protein, mushrooms are particularly useful for plant-based diets. Mushrooms also help to burn fat in the body because their nutrients help to regulate glucose levels in the blood. Their excellent nutritional value will keep you energized and allow you to workout for longer.

Is it safe?

Hen-of-the-woods, oyster, and sulphur shelf mushrooms are safe, delicious, and nutritious wild varieties prized by mushroom hunters. While these and many other mushrooms are safe to consume, eating varieties like the death cap, false morels, and Conocybe filaris can cause serious adverse health effects and even death.

N

N-acetylcysteine (NAC) (see COVID-19)

N-acetyl cysteine is an antioxidant that might play a role in preventing cancer. As a drug, it's used by healthcare providers to treat acetaminophen (Tylenol) poisoning. It works by binding the poisonous forms of acetaminophen that are formed in the liver.

Does it work?

N-acetyl cysteine is an antioxidant that might play a role in preventing cancer. As a drug, it's used by healthcare providers to treat acetaminophen (Tylenol) poisoning. It works by binding the poisonous forms of acetaminophen that are formed in the liver.

Is it safe?

When taken by mouth: N-acetyl cysteine is likely safe for most adults. N-acetyl cysteine is an FDA-approved prescription drug. It can cause side effects such as dry mouth, nausea, vomiting, and diarrhea. It has an unpleasant odor that some people find hard to tolerate.

Nicotinamide Riboside (NR)

Nicotinamide riboside is a pyridine-nucleoside similar to vitamin B_3, functioning as a precursor to nicotinamide adenine dinucleotide or NAD+.

Does it work?

Taking nicotinamide riboside can help raise low NAD+ levels. People use nicotinamide riboside for anti-aging effects, high cholesterol, high blood pressure, Alzheimer disease, obesity, and many other purposes, but there is no good scientific evidence to support these uses.

Is it safe?

Nicotinamide riboside is likely safe with few if any side effects. In human studies, taking 1,000–2,000 mg per day had no harmful effects.

Niacin

Niacin, or vitamin B3, is a water-soluble B vitamin found naturally in some foods, added to foods, and sold as a supplement. The two most common forms of niacin in food and supplements are nicotinic acid and nicotinamide. The body can also convert tryptophan an amino acid to nicotinamide.

Does it work?

Niacin works by lowering both your low-density lipoprotein (LDL) or "bad" cholesterol and other fatty substances (triglycerides) in your blood and raising your high-density lipoprotein (HDL) or "good" cholesterol. Niacin works with exercise and a healthy diet to improve your cholesterol levels.

Is it safe?

When taken orally in appropriate amounts, niacin appears to be safe. High doses of niacin available via prescription can cause: Severe skin flushing combined with dizziness. Rapid heartbeat.

Nitric Oxide

Nitric oxide is a compound in the body that causes blood vessels to widen and stimulates the release of certain hormones, such as insulin and human growth hormone. Nitric oxide supplements are a category of supplements that includes L-citrulline and L-arginine.

Does it work?

Circulatory system : Nitric oxide appears to help your body dilate and constrict your blood vessels. This can improve your blood pressure and therefore your heart health. Exercise and muscle performance : Nitric oxide may be correlated to a slight improvement in physical performance.

Is it safe?

Nitric Oxide is extremely toxic by inhalation, and symptoms of over-exposure may not become apparent for up to 72 hours. The gas is an oxidizer and will support and enhance combustion. Emergency responders must protect themselves from inhalation. A water spray can be used to control and direct a release.

Noni

Morinda citrifolia is a fruit-bearing tree in the coffee family, Rubiaceae. Its native range extends across Southeast Asia and Australasia, and was spread across the Pacific by Polynesian sailors. The species is now cultivated throughout the tropics and widely naturalized.

Does it work?

People use noni for cancer, high blood pressure, athletic performance, aging skin, diabetes, and many other conditions, but there is no good scientific evidence to support these uses. The US FDA has issued multiple warnings to noni manufacturers for making health claims that aren't supported by research.

Is it safe?

Although there isn't a daily recommended intake of noni juice, studies show that drinking up to 750 milliliters, or just over 25 ounces, of noni juice per day is safe. In fact, noni juice is considered just as safe as other common fruit juices.

Nootropics

Nootropics, or "smart drugs," are a class of substances that can boost brain performance. They are sometimes called cognition enhancers or memory enhancing substances. Prescription nootropics are medications that have stimulant effects.

Does it work?

Some small studies show that some nootropic supplements can affect the brain. But there is a lack of evidence from large, controlled studies to show that some of these supplements consistently work and are completely safe.

Is it safe?

Conclusion. Nootropics are safe if you have an awareness of risks and how to avoid them. There is always a risk that you will have edge-case side effects. To avoid these, start with small dosages and do your research beforehand.

O

Olive

Olive, (Olea europaea), subtropical broad-leaved evergreen tree (family Oleaceae) and its edible fruit. The olive fruit and its oil are key elements in the cuisine of the Mediterranean and are popular outside the region. olive. Related Topics: evergreen olive.

Does it work?
Olives have a low calorie density and are a good source of healthy fats, two factors that may boost weight loss by helping keep you full and replacing less healthy fats in your diet.

Is it safe?
Up to 1 liter of extra-virgin olive oil weekly has been used safely as part of a Mediterranean-style diet for up to 5.8 years. Olive oil is usually well-tolerated. It might cause nausea in a small number of people. Olive leaf extract is possibly safe when used appropriately.

Omega-3 Fatty Acids
Omega-3 fatty acids are found in foods, such as fish and flaxseed, and in dietary supplements, such as fish oil. The three main omega-3 fatty acids are alpha-linolenic acid (ALA), eicosapentaenoic acid (EPA), and docosahexaenoic acid (DHA). ALA is found mainly in plant oils such as flaxseed, soybean, and canola oils.

Does it work?
They also bind to receptors in cells that regulate genetic function. Likely due to these effects, omega-3 fats have been shown to help prevent heart disease and stroke, may help control lupus, eczema, and rheumatoid arthritis, and may play protective roles in cancer and other conditions.

Is it safe?
Side effects of omega-3 supplements are usually mild. They include unpleasant taste, bad breath, bad-smelling sweat, headache, and gastrointestinal symptoms such as heartburn, nausea, and diarrhea. Several large studies have linked higher blood levels of long-chain omega-3s with higher risks of prostate cancer.

Omega-6 Fatty Acids

Omega-6 fatty acids are a type of polyunsaturated fat found in vegetable oils, nuts and seeds. When eaten in moderation and in place of saturated fats, omega-6 fatty acids can be good for the heart and appear to protect against heart disease.

Does it work?
Along with omega-3 fatty acids, omega-6 fatty acids play a crucial role in brain function, and normal growth and development. As a type of polyunsaturated fatty acid (PUFA), omega-6s help stimulate skin and hair growth, maintain bone health, regulate metabolism, and maintain the reproductive system.

Is it safe?
Omega-6 fatty acids are LIKELY SAFE when consumed by adults and children over the age of 12 months as part of the diet in amounts between 5% and 10% of daily calories.

Omega-7 Fatty Acids
Omega-7 fatty acids are a class of unsaturated fatty acids in which the site of unsaturation is seven carbon atoms from the end of the carbon chain. The two most common omega-7 fatty acids in nature are palmitoleic acid and vaccenic acid. They are widely used in cosmetics due to their moisturizing properties.

Does it work?
Omega-7 fats are not essential fatty acids in humans as they can be made endogenously. Diets rich in omega-7 fatty acids have been shown to have beneficial health effects, such as increasing levels of HDL cholesterol and lowering levels of LDL cholesterol.

Is it safe?
Omega-7 fats are not essential fatty acids in humans as they can be made endogenously. Diets rich in omega-7 fatty acids have been shown to have beneficial health effects, such as increasing levels of HDL cholesterol and lowering levels of LDL cholesterol.

Okg Ornithine

Ornithine ketoglutarate is a salt made from the amino acid ornithine and the glutamine precursor alpha-ketoglutarate. People use it as a medicine.

Does it work?
Ornithine ketoglutarate might change the way amino acids, the building blocks of protein, are used in the body. It also increases insulin, a hormone that regulates the amount of sugar in the blood.

Is it safe?
Ornithine ketoglutarate is possibly safe in children and adults when given intravenously or in adults when taken by mouth with appropriate medical supervision.

Oregano
Oregano (Origanum vulgare) is an herb used to flavor foods. It is considered safe in common food amounts, but has little evidence of health benefits. Oregano has olive-green leaves and purple flowers. It is closely related to other herbs, including mint, thyme, marjoram, and basil.

Does it work?
Oregano contains chemicals that might help reduce cough. Oregano also might help with digestion and with fighting against some bacteria and viruses. People use oregano for wound healing, parasite infections, and many other conditions, but there is no good scientific evidence to support these uses.

Is it safe?
Experts agree that oregano is safe when used for its intended purpose -- adding flavor to food. Oregano's safety for medicinal purposes is not known. Due to some of its properties, a few things should be kept in mind when taking oregano or oregano oil in medicinal amounts.

Osteoarthritis
Osteoarthritis is the most common form of arthritis, affecting millions of people worldwide. It occurs when the protective cartilage that cushions the ends of the bones wears down over time. Although osteoarthritis can damage any joint, the disorder most commonly affects joints in your hands, knees, hips and spine.

Does it work?
Osteoarthritis symptoms can usually be managed, although the damage to joints can't be reversed. Staying active, maintaining a healthy weight and receiving certain treatments might slow progression of the disease and help improve pain and joint function.

Is it safe?
Because of pain, muscle weakness, and joint stiffness, osteoarthritis may cause trouble with balance. And as osteoarthritis progresses, tasks like climbing stairs, getting into the tub, and even walking across the room can become a challenge, leading to a real risk of falling.

P

Pantothenic Acid
Pantothenic acid (also known as vitamin B5) is an essential nutrient that is naturally present in some foods, added to others, and available as a dietary supplement. The main function of this water-soluble B vitamin is in the synthesis of coenzyme A (CoA) and acyl carrier protein

Does it work?
Vitamin B5, also called pantothenic acid, is one of the most important vitamins for human life. It's necessary for making blood cells, and it helps you convert the food you eat into energy. Vitamin B5 is one of eight B vitamins. All B vitamins help you convert the protein, carbohydrates, and fats you eat into energy.

Is it safe?
When taken by mouth: Pantothenic acid is likely safe for most people. The recommended amount for adults is 5 mg per day. Larger amounts (up to 1 gram) seem to be safe for most people. But taking larger amounts increases the chance of side effects such as diarrhea.

Papaya
The papaya, papaw, or pawpaw is the plant Carica papaya, one of the 22 accepted species in the genus Carica of the family Caricaceae. It was first domesticated in Mesoamerica, within

modern-day southern Mexico and Central America. In 2020, India produced 43% of the world supply of papayas.

Does it work?

Unripe papaya contains a chemical called papain. Papain breaks down proteins, carbohydrates, and fats. But papain is changed in the stomach, so it's not clear if it's effective as medicine when taken by mouth. Papaya also contains a chemical called carpain, which seems to be able to kill certain parasites and might affect the central nervous system.

Is it safe?

Papaya (Carica papaya) is a tropical tree. Its ripe fruit is considered safe, but unripe papaya fruit contains papain and can damage the esophagus. Unripe papaya contains a chemical called papain. Papain breaks down proteins, carbohydrates, and fats.

Phenibut

Phenibut (beta-phenyl-gamma-aminobutyric acid HCl) is a neuropsychotropic drug that was discovered and introduced into clinical practice in Russia in the 1960s. It has anxiolytic and nootropic (cognition enhancing) effects. It acts as a GABA-mimetic, primarily at GABA(B) and, to some extent, at GABA(A) receptors.

Does it work?

Phenibut might decrease anxiety and have other effects on the body, but most research on phenibut has been published in Russia. People use phenibut for anxiety, alcohol use disorder, insomnia, depression, stress, and many other conditions, but there is no good scientific evidence to support these uses.

Is it safe?

The current systematic review provides evidence that, at therapeutic doses, phenibut is safe and well tolerated with minor adverse effects, but questions regarding the quality of phenibut obtained online and the contribution of alcohol and other drug abuse to phenibut dependence and intoxication remain open.

Passion Flower

Passiflora incarnata, commonly known as maypop, purple passionflower, true passionflower, wild apricot, and wild passion vine, is a fast-growing perennial vine with climbing or trailing stems. A member of the passionflower genus Passiflora, the maypop has large, intricate flowers with prominent styles and stamens.

Does it work?
Studies of people with generalized anxiety disorder show that passionflower is as effective as the drug oxazepam (Serax) for treating symptoms. Passionflower didn't work as quickly as oxazepam (day 7 compared to day 4). However, it produced less impairment on job performance than oxazepam.

Is it safe?
When taken by mouth: Passion flower is likely safe for most people when used as a flavoring in foods. It's possibly safe when taken as a tea for 7 nights, or as a medicine for up to 8 weeks. It may cause side effects such as drowsiness, dizziness, and confusion.

Pau d'Arco
Pau d'arco (Tabebuia impetiginosa) is a tree that is native to the Amazon. Its bark and wood have been used for many conditions, but with little evidence. The pau d'arco tree is used by native peoples in the regions where it grows for making hunting bows.

Does it work?
Pau d'arco is a supplement made from the inner bark of a tropical tree. While test-tube and animal studies suggest that this bark helps treat certain infections and reduces inflammation, studies in humans are lacking. Therefore, the effectiveness and safety of pau d'arco extract remain largely unknown.

Is it safe?
When taken by mouth: Pau d'arco is possibly unsafe. In high doses, a chemical found in pau d'arco can cause severe nausea, vomiting, diarrhea, dizziness, and internal bleeding. The safety of pau d'arco in typical doses is not known.

Pycnogenol

Pycnogenol is a compound of natural chemicals. It comes from the bark of a European pine tree.

Does it work?
Pycnogenol seems to help with asthma and allergies. Early research shows that taking it at least 5 weeks before the start of allergy season seems to lessen symptoms. In a small/preliminary study of kids with asthma, pycnogenol helped improve symptoms. It also lessened the amount of asthma medication they needed.

Is it safe?
Pycnogenol is POSSIBLY SAFE when taken by mouth in doses of 50 mg to 450 mg daily for up to one year, and when applied to the skin as a cream for up to 7 days or as a powder for up to 6 weeks. Pycnogenol can cause dizziness, gut problems, headache, and mouth ulcers.

Phytonutrients
Phytonutrients are natural compounds found in plant foods such as vegetables, fruit, whole grain products and legumes. These plant compounds have beneficial effects working with other essential nutrients to promote good health.

Does it work?
Phytonutrients aren't essential for keeping you alive, unlike the vitamins and minerals that plant foods contain. But when you eat or drink phytonutrients, they may help prevent disease and keep your body working properly. More than 25,000 phytonutrients are found in plant foods.

Is it safe?
Phytonutrients aren't essential for keeping you alive, unlike the vitamins and minerals that plant foods contain. But when you eat or drink phytonutrients, they may help prevent disease and keep your body working properly. More than 25,000 phytonutrients are found in plant foods.

PC-SPES
PC-SPES is a supplement consisting of eight herbs: reishi mushroom, baikal skullcap, rabdosia, dyer's woad, chrysanthemum, saw palmetto, Panax ginseng, and licorice.

Laboratory studies suggested it may have anticancer effects, particularly against prostate cancer.

Does it work?
There is evidence from both laboratory and animal studies to suggest that PC-SPES had some effect in inhibiting prostate cancer cell growth and prostate-specific antigen (PSA) expression, but it is not known whether these results were caused by adulterants such as diethylstilbestrol, which is an estrogenic compound.

Is it safe?
Each herb used in PC-SPES has been reported to have anti-inflammatory, antioxidant, or anticarcinogenic properties. PC-SPES was recalled and withdrawn from the market because certain batches were contaminated with Food and Drug Administration–controlled prescription drugs.

Peppermint Oil
Peppermint oil is derived from the peppermint plant -- a cross between water mint and spearmint -- that thrives in Europe and North America. Peppermint oil is commonly used as flavoring in foods and beverages and as a fragrance in soaps and cosmetics.

Does it work?
While some of the proposed benefits of peppermint oil come from anecdotal evidence, research suggests peppermint oil may be beneficial for IBS and other digestive conditions, as well as pain relief. Peppermint oil is generally safe, but it can be toxic when taken in very large doses.

Is it safe?
Peppermint oil appears to be safe when taken orally (by mouth) or applied topically in the doses commonly used. Peppermint oil has been safely used in many clinical trials. Possible side effects of peppermint oil taken orally include heartburn, nausea, abdominal pain, and dry mouth.

Phytoestrogens
Phytoestrogens (plant oestrogens) are substances that occur naturally in plants. They have a similar chemical structure to our own body's oestrogen (one of the main female

hormones), and are able to bind to the same receptors that our own oestrogen does.

Does it work?
Phytoestrogens are plant-based compounds that mimic estrogen in the body. They have been found to be beneficial in combatting symptoms and conditions caused by estrogen deficiency. This may be of particular benefit to premenopausal and post-menopausal women. Phytoestrogens may also play a role in fighting cancer.

Is it safe?
In fact, phytoestrogens are classified as endocrine disruptors. These are chemicals that may interfere with the body's hormonal system when consumed at a sufficiently high dose. However, there's not much evidence that phytoestrogens have harmful effects in humans.

Performance: Exercise and Athletic (see Exercise and Athletic Performance)
A performance is an act of staging or presenting a play, concert, or other form of entertainment. It is also defined as the action or process of carrying out or accomplishing an action, task, or function.

Phosphorus
Phosphorus is a component of bones, teeth, DNA, and RNA [1]. In the form of phospholipids, phosphorus is also a component of cell membrane structure and of the body's key energy source, ATP. Many proteins and sugars in the body are phosphorylated.

Does it work?
The main function of phosphorus is in the formation of bones and teeth. It plays an important role in how the body uses carbohydrates and fats. It is also needed for the body to make protein for the growth, maintenance, and repair of cells and tissues.

Is it safe?
High phosphorus levels can cause damage to your body. Extra phosphorus causes body changes that pull calcium out of your bones, making them weak. High phosphorus and

calcium levels also lead to dangerous calcium deposits in blood vessels, lungs, eyes, and heart.

Pomegranate

The pomegranate is a fruit-bearing deciduous shrub in the family Lythraceae, subfamily Punicoideae, that grows between 5 and 10 m tall. The pomegranate was originally described throughout the Mediterranean region.

Does it work?

Pomegranate juice is in the running as the most heart-healthy juice. It appears to protect the heart and arteries. Small studies have shown that the juice improves blood flow and keeps the arteries from becoming stiff and thick. It may also slow the growth of plaque and buildup of cholesterol in the arteries.

Is it safe?

Pomegranate extract may also be safe. Pomegranate root, stem, and peel may not be safe when consumed in large amounts because they contain substances that can have harmful effects. Pomegranate usually doesn't have side effects, but digestive tract symptoms, especially diarrhea, may occur in a small number of people.

Pelargonium Sidoides

Pelargonium sidoides is a plant native to South Africa. Its common names include African geranium and South African geranium.

Does it work?

It is used in Europe to treat the common cold and bronchitis. In laboratory studies, this herb was shown to kill bacteria, viruses, and stimulate the immune system. Human studies show that it can reduce the symptoms of common cold and bronchitis.

Is it safe?

The safety of pelargonium remedies is largely untested. Commonly cited side effects include stomach upset, nausea, heartburn, or worsening respiratory symptoms. Pelargonium contains a substance known as coumarin that acts as an anticoagulant (blood thinner).

Potassium
Potassium is an essential mineral that is needed by all tissues in the body. It is sometimes referred to as an electrolyte because it carries a small electrical charge that activates various cell and nerve functions. Potassium is found naturally in many foods and as a supplement.

Does it work?
It is a type of electrolyte. It helps your nerves to function and muscles to contract. It helps your heartbeat stay regular. It also helps move nutrients into cells and waste products out of cells.

Is it safe?
At normal doses, potassium is fairly safe. It may cause an upset stomach. Some people have allergies to potassium supplements.

Primary Mitochondrial Disorders
Primary mitochondrial myopathies (PMM) are a group of disorders that are associated with changes in genetic material (e.g. depletions, deletions, or mutations) found within the DNA of mitochondria (mtDNA) or with genes outside the mitochondria (nuclear DNA), affecting predominantly the skeletal muscle.

Probiotics
Probiotics are microorganisms in foods, such as some yogurts, and some dietary supplements that help maintain or restore beneficial bacteria in your digestive tract.

Does it work?
It's unclear whether probiotic supplements have any effect on weight or body fat.

Is it safe?
Probiotics are safe in healthy people but may cause gas or other gastrointestinal problems.

Prebiotics
Prebiotics are compounds in food that induce the growth or activity of beneficial microorganisms such as bacteria and fungi. The most common example is in the gastrointestinal

tract, where prebiotics can alter the composition of organisms in the gut microbiome.

Does it work?
Prebiotics are special plant fibers that help healthy bacteria grow in your gut. This makes your digestive system work better.

Is it safe?
Prebiotics have a long history of safe use and have been known for their health benefits in humans, including an increase in the bioavailability of minerals, modulation of the immune system, prevention of gastrointestinal (GI) infections, modification of inflammatory conditions, regulation of metabolic disorders.

Propolis
Propolis or bee glue is a resinous mixture that honey bees produce by mixing saliva and beeswax with exudate gathered from tree buds, sap flows, or other botanical sources. It is used as a sealant for unwanted open spaces in the beehive.

Does it work?
Propolis has a special compound called pinocembrin, a flavonoid that acts as an antifungal. These anti-inflammatory and antimicrobial properties make propolis helpful in wound healing. One study found that propolis can help people who have had traumatic burns heal faster by speeding up new healthy cell growth.

Is it safe?
When taken by mouth: Propolis is possibly safe when used appropriately. It can cause allergic reactions, especially in people who are allergic to other bee products. Lozenges containing propolis can cause irritation and mouth ulcers. When applied to the skin: Propolis is possibly safe when used appropriately.

Protein Powder (see Exercise and Athletic Performance)
Protein is an important part of a healthy diet. Proteins are made up of chemical 'building blocks' called amino acids. Your body uses amino acids to build and repair muscles and bones

and to make hormones and enzymes. They can also be used as an energy source.

Does it work?
As mentioned before, protein shakes provide amino acids that are easily absorbed by your body. Researchers believe that their intake increases amino acid levels in the bloodstream, which in turn triggers a more significant response for muscle synthesis.

Is it safe?
Protein powders are generally recognized as safe, although you may experience digestive side effects if you consume large amounts of protein powder. If you're lactose intolerant or otherwise sensitive to lactose, dairy-based protein powder may lead to stomach upset, bloating, and gas.

Psyllium (blond)
Psyllium, or ispaghula, is the common name used for several members of the plant genus Plantago whose seeds are used commercially for the production of mucilage. Psyllium is mainly used as a dietary fiber to relieve symptoms of both constipation and mild diarrhea, and occasionally as a food thickener.

Does it work?
Many well-designed studies have shown that psyllium relieves constipation. When combined with water, it swells and produces more bulk, which stimulates the intestines to contract and helps speed the passage of stool through the digestive tract. Psyllium is widely used as a laxative in Asia, Europe, and North America.

Is it safe?
There's no evidence that daily use of fiber supplements such as psyllium (Metamucil, Konsyl, others) or methylcellulose (Citrucel) is harmful. Fiber has a number of health benefits, including normalizing bowel function and preventing constipation.

Pyruvate (see Weight Loss)
Pyruvate is naturally present in your body. Pyruvate in weight-loss supplements is claimed to increase fat breakdown,

reduce body weight and body fat, and improve exercise performance.

Does it work?
Pyruvate in supplements might help you lose a small amount of weight.

Is it safe?
Pyruvate seems to be safe (at up to 30 g a day for 6 weeks). It can cause diarrhea, gas, bloating, and rumbling noises in the intestines due to gas.

Q

Quercetin (see Exercise and Athletic Performance)
Quercetin is a plant pigment (flavonoid). It's found in many plants and foods, such as red wine, onions, green tea, apples, and berries. Quercetin has antioxidant and anti-inflammatory effects that might help reduce swelling, kill cancer cells, control blood sugar, and help prevent heart disease.

Does it work?
The current study shows that intake of quercetin may improve endurance exercise performance but may not reduce the body fat percent. Thus, more studies with longer periods of supplementation and larger doses that may increase quercetin bioactive effects are necessary.

Is it safe?
Quercetin is generally considered safe. Side effects may include headache and upset stomach. Preliminary evidence suggests that a byproduct of quercetin can lead to a loss of protein function. Very high doses of quercetin may damage the kidneys.

R

Raspberry Ketones
Raspberry ketone is a natural phenolic compound that is the primary aroma compound of red raspberries.

Does it work?
It's believed that raspberry ketone might increase metabolism, increase how quickly the body burns fat, and

reduce appetite. But evidence in humans is limited. Raspberry ketone is also found in kiwifruit, peaches, grapes, apples, other berries, rhubarb, and the bark of yew, maple, and pine trees.

Is it safe?
Raspberry ketones in food and cosmetics are generally considered safe. But no one knows what short- or long-term effect raspberry ketone supplements could have on your overall health. No study has been done to document potential side effects. There are also no studies that look at potential drug or food interactions.

Red Clover
Trifolium pratense, the red clover, is a herbaceous species of flowering plant in the bean family Fabaceae, native to Europe, Western Asia, and northwest Africa, but planted and naturalized in many other regions.

Does it work?
Some research has found taking 40–80 mg of red clover daily may help reduce severe menopausal hot flashes. However, beyond this, little evidence supports using red clover to treat other health conditions. Though it has a good safety profile, some side effects include nausea, vomiting, headache, and vaginal spotting.

Is it safe?
It is possibly safe to take red clover in doses that provide up to 80 mg of isoflavones daily for up to 2 years. It's usually well-tolerated, but might cause muscle aches, nausea, and vaginal bleeding (spotting) in some people. When applied to the skin: Red clover is possibly safe when used for up to 4 weeks.

Resveratrol
Resveratrol is a stilbenoid, a type of natural phenol, and a phytoalexin produced by several plants in response to injury or when the plant is under attack by pathogens, such as bacteria or fungi. Sources of resveratrol in food include the skin of grapes, blueberries, raspberries, mulberries, and peanuts.

Does it work?
Resveratrol might have many effects in the body, including expanding blood vessels and reducing blood clotting. It may

also decrease pain and swelling, reduce levels of sugar in the blood, and help the body fight against disease.

Is it safe?
When you get resveratrol in the amount naturally found in foods, it is generally considered safe. It could cause a reaction in those who are allergic to grapes or wine. People who have health conditions like bleeding disorders should not take resveratrol without talking to a doctor first.

Rheumatoid Arthritis
Rheumatoid arthritis, or RA, is an autoimmune and inflammatory disease, which means that your immune system attacks healthy cells in your body by mistake, causing inflammation (painful swelling) in the affected parts of the body. RA mainly attacks the joints, usually many joints at once.

Does it work?
There is no cure for rheumatoid arthritis. But clinical studies indicate that remission of symptoms is more likely when treatment begins early with medications known as disease-modifying antirheumatic drugs (DMARDs).

Is it safe?
Rheumatoid arthritis (RA) has many physical and social consequences and can lower quality of life. It can cause pain, disability, and premature death. Premature heart disease. People with RA are also at a higher risk for developing other chronic diseases such as heart disease and diabetes.

Rhodiola
Rhodiola rosea is a perennial flowering plant in the family Crassulaceae. It grows naturally in wild Arctic regions of Europe, Asia, and North America, and can be propagated as a groundcover.

Does it work?
According to current research findings, rhodiola may be effective for improving symptoms of stress, fatigue, or depression when taken in doses ranging from 400–600 mg per day taken in single or divided doses.

Is it safe?

Rhodiola rosea extract WS® 1375 was safe and generally well tolerated. Adverse events were mostly of mild intensity and no serious adverse events were reported. Rhodiola extract at a dose of 200 mg twice daily for 4 weeks is safe and effective in improving life-stress symptoms to a clinically relevant degree.

Royal Jelly
Royal jelly is a milky secretion produced by worker honeybees. It typically contains about 60% to 70% water, 12% to 15% proteins, 10% to 16% sugar, 3% to 6% fats, and 2% to 3% vitamins, salts, and amino acids. Its composition varies depending on geography and climate.

Does it work?
There is very little scientific information available about the effects of royal jelly in people. In animals, royal jelly seems to have some activity against tumors and the development of "hardening of the arteries."

Is it safe?
When taken by mouth: Royal jelly is possibly safe for most people when taken at appropriate doses. Doses up to 4.8 grams per day for up to 1 year have been used safely. In people with asthma or allergies, royal jelly might cause serious allergic reactions.

Riboflavin
Riboflavin, also known as vitamin B_2, is a vitamin found in food and sold as a dietary supplement. It is essential to the formation of two major coenzymes, flavin mononucleotide and flavin adenine dinucleotide.

Does it work?
Vitamin B2, also called riboflavin, is one of 8 B vitamins. All B vitamins help the body to convert food (carbohydrates) into fuel (glucose), which is used to produce energy. These B vitamins, often referred to as B-complex vitamins, also help the body metabolize fats and protein.

Is it safe?
Relatively nontoxic, riboflavin is considered safe at high doses because excess is disposed of through the urinary tract. There may be some side effects from taking higher doses of B2,

though. "Some people notice their urine turning yellow-orange in color and having diarrhea when taken in higher doses.

Ribose (see Exercise and Athletic Performance)
Ribose is a sugar that is naturally produced by the body from food. It is a natural part of DNA and RNA and is required for many processes in the body. Supplemental ribose might prevent muscle fatigue in people with certain genetic disorders that affect energy production by the body.

Does it work?
Ribose is a sugar that is naturally produced by the body from food. It is a natural part of DNA and RNA and is required for many processes in the body. Supplemental ribose might prevent muscle fatigue in people with certain genetic disorders that affect energy production by the body.

Is it safe?
When taken by mouth: Ribose is commonly consumed in foods. It is likely safe for most people when taken for up to 1 month as medicine. It can cause some side effects including diarrhea, stomach discomfort, nausea, headache, and low blood sugar.

Red Yeast Rice
Red yeast rice is made by culturing rice with various strains of the yeast Monascus purpureus. Some preparations of red yeast rice are used in food products in Chinese cuisine, including Peking duck. Others have been sold as dietary supplements to lower blood levels of cholesterol and related lipids.

Does it work?
Studies have shown that certain red yeast rice products that contain statin can significantly lower levels of total cholesterol and specifically LDL, or "bad" cholesterol. One showed that taking 2.4 grams per day reduced LDL levels by 22% and total cholesterol by 16% in 12 weeks.

Is it safe?
Caution. Red yeast rice is capable of lowering blood cholesterol levels and total blood cholesterol levels. While the supplement is generally considered safe, it might carry the

same potential side effects as statin cholesterol drugs. Red yeast rice might cost less than a statin.

Rose Hips
The rose hip or rosehip, also called rose haw and rose hep, is the accessory fruit of the various species of rose plant. It is typically red to orange, but ranges from dark purple to black in some species.

Does it work?
Overall, research suggests that rose hip is beneficial for people with osteoarthritis. Most research shows that taking a specific rose hip product (Hyben Vital) twice daily for 3-4 months reduces pain and stiffness and improves function in people with osteoarthritis.

Is it safe?
Rosehip is generally considered safe when taken by mouth and used as directed. Reported side effects have included: Diarrhea. Fatigue.

S

S-adenosyl-L-Methionine (SAMe)
S-Adenosyl methionine is a common cosubstrate involved in methyl group transfers, transsulfuration, and aminopropylation. Although these anabolic reactions occur throughout the body, most SAM-e is produced and consumed in the liver.

Does it work?
SAMe helps produce and regulate hormones and maintain cell membranes. A synthetic version of SAMe is available as a dietary supplement in the U.S. In some countries in Europe, SAMe is a prescription drug.

Is it safe?
More like a vitamin than a drug, SAM-e is a natural metabolite that the body needs more of as we age or if we become ill. SAM-e is generally safe and evidence-based for the treatment of depression. It is also a promising neuroprotectant and may be helpful in treating ADHD.

Supplements Androstenedione

Androstenedione is also sold as an oral supplement, that is being utilized to increase testosterone levels. Simply known as "andro" by athletes, it is commonly touted as a natural alternative to anabolic steroids.

Does it work?
Several studies have reported that supplementation with 200–300 mg/day androstenedione can produce acute and chronic increases in total and free testosterone concentrations, whereas others have reported no changes, in younger (<40 years) and middle aged (☐40 years) men.

Is it safe?
Androstenedione is possibly unsafe for most people when taken by mouth. Some side effects experienced by men include reduced sperm production, shrunken testicles, painful or prolonged erections, breast development, behavioral changes, heart disease, and others.

Sports Drinks
Sports drinks, also known as electrolyte drinks, are functional beverages whose stated purpose is to help athletes replace water, electrolytes, and energy before, during and especially after training or competition, though their effects on performance in sports and exercise has been questioned.

Does it work?
Six of the studies showed that sports drinks benefited exercise performance. However, all participants were trained athletes performing intense exercise. One study in trained cyclists found that a sports drink improved performance by about 2% during one hour of intense cycling, compared to a placebo.

Is it safe?
Although sports drinks can improve the performance of athletes during several types of exercise, they are probably unnecessary for most people. If you choose to drink these beverages, it is important not to overconsume them.

Saccharomyces Boulardii
Saccharomyces boulardii is a yeast believed to be a strain of Saccharomyces cerevisiae. It is likely effective for treating

certain types of diarrhea. Saccharomyces boulardii is called a "probiotic," a friendly organism that helps to fight off "bad" organisms that might cause diseases.

Does it work?
Saccharomyces boulardii is a yeast believed to be a strain of Saccharomyces cerevisiae. It is likely effective for treating certain types of diarrhea. Saccharomyces boulardii is called a "probiotic," a friendly organism that helps to fight off "bad" organisms that might cause diseases.

Is it safe?
Saccharomyces boulardii is likely safe for most adults when taken by mouth for up to 15 months. It can cause gas in some people. Rarely, it might cause fungal infections that can spread through the bloodstream to the entire body (fungemia).

Sage
Sage is commonly used as a spice to flavor foods. As medicine, common sage extract has most often been used by adults in doses of 280-1500 mg by mouth daily for up to 12 weeks. Sage is also used in essential oils, creams, ointments, sprays, and mouth rinses.

Does it work?
Some very preliminary evidence suggests that sage might help improve symptoms of menopause, such as night sweats or hot flashes. Sage is available as a tea, essential oil, and oral supplement. Only the supplement form of sage has been shown to be helpful for menopausal symptoms.

Is it safe?
When consumed for culinary purposes, sage is considered safe in adults and children. By contrast, when used for medicinal purposes, sage or sage extract can be harmful if overused or used for a long period of time.

Sulfur
Sulfur is a chemical element with the symbol S and atomic number 16. It is abundant, multivalent and nonmetallic. Under normal conditions, sulfur atoms form cyclic octatomic molecules with a chemical formula S_8. Elemental sulfur is a bright yellow, crystalline solid at room temperature.

Does it work?
It is the third most abundant mineral in the human body. Sulfur seems to have antibacterial effects against the bacteria that cause acne. It also might help promote the loosening and shedding of skin. This is believed to help treat skin conditions such as seborrheic dermatitis or acne.

Is it safe?
Sulfur is low in toxicity to people. However, ingesting too much sulfur may cause a burning sensation or diarrhea. Breathing in sulfur dust can irritate the airways or cause coughing. It can also be irritating to the skin and eyes.

Supplements for Skin Care
Skin care is the range of practices that support skin integrity, enhance its appearance and relieve skin conditions. They can include nutrition, avoidance of excessive sun exposure and appropriate use of emollients.

Does it work?
There is no research showing that supplements play a role in your skin's health when you're an otherwise healthy person with no vitamin deficiencies.

Is it safe?
Most emollients can be used safely and effectively with no side effects. However, burning, stinging, redness, or irritation may occur.

Saw Palmetto
Saw palmetto extract is an extract of the fruit of the saw palmetto. It is marketed as a treatment for benign prostatic hyperplasia, but there is no clinical evidence that it is effective for this purpose.

Does it work?
Some studies show that saw palmetto is as effective in treating symptoms as finasteride (Proscar) without side effects, such as loss of libido. Other studies suggest that saw palmetto may actually shrink the size of the prostate gland.

Is it safe?
When taken by mouth: Saw palmetto is likely safe when used for up to 3 years. Side effects are usually mild and might

include dizziness, headache, nausea, and diarrhea. When given rectally: Saw palmetto is possibly safe when used for up to 30 days. It's unknown if it is safe to use for longer periods of time.

Selenium

It is found naturally in foods or as a supplement. Selenium is an essential component of various enzymes and proteins, called selenoproteins, that help to make DNA and protect against cell damage and infections; these proteins are also involved in reproduction and the metabolism of thyroid hormones.

Does it work?

Selenium has attracted attention because of its antioxidant properties. Antioxidants protect cells from damage. Evidence that selenium supplements may reduce the odds of prostate cancer has been mixed, but most studies suggest there is no real benefit.

Is it safe?

When taken by mouth: Selenium is likely safe when taken in doses less than 400 mcg daily, short-term. But selenium is possibly unsafe when taken in high doses or for a long time. Taking doses above 400 mcg daily can increase the risk of developing selenium toxicity.

Sulforaphane

Sulforaphane is a compound within the isothiocyanate group of organosulfur compounds. It is obtained from cruciferous vegetables such as broccoli, Brussels sprouts, and cabbages.

Does it work?

Some studies have shown that sulforaphane blocks mutations in DNA that lead to cancer. It may slow tumor growth. Sulforaphane has been shown to reduce the ability of cancerous cells to multiply. That means it may slow tumor growth or reduce its ability to spread to other parts of your body.

Is it safe?

When taken by mouth: Sulforaphane is likely safe when used in the amounts found in foods. It is possibly safe when taken in medicinal amounts. Sulforaphane and sulforaphane-rich broccoli extract products have been used safely for up to 6 months.

Senna
Senna is the fruit (pod) or leaf of the plant Senna alexandrina. It is approved in the US as a laxative for short-term treatment of constipation. Senna contains many chemicals called sennosides. Sennosides irritate the lining of the bowel, which causes a laxative effect.

Does it work?
Senna works by encouraging the muscles in your bowel to move stools through your body. This helps you to go to the toilet. It usually has an effect within 8-12 hours.

Is it safe?
When taken by mouth: Senna is likely safe for most adults when used for up to 1 week. Senna is an FDA-approved nonprescription (OTC) medicine. It can cause some side effects including stomach discomfort, cramps, and diarrhea.

Shark Cartilage
Shark cartilage is the tissue that provides support for fins in sharks (Squalus acanthias). It mainly comes from sharks caught in the Pacific Ocean.

Does it work?
Shark cartilage can increase the activity of the immune system. Some medications, such as those used after a transplant, decrease the activity of the immune system. Taking shark cartilage along with these medications might decrease the effects of these medications.

Is it safe?
When taken by mouth: Shark cartilage is possibly safe when used for up to 40 months. It can cause a bad taste in the mouth, nausea, vomiting, stomach upset, and constipation. When applied to the skin: Shark cartilage is possibly safe when used for up to 8 weeks.

Slippery Elm
Ulmus rubra, the slippery elm, is a species of elm native to eastern North America, ranging from southeast North Dakota,

east to Maine and southern Quebec, south to northernmost Florida, and west to eastern Texas, where it thrives in moist uplands, although it will also grow in dry, intermediate soils.

Does it work?
The inner bark contains chemicals that can increase mucous secretion, which might be helpful for stomach and intestinal problems. People use slippery elm for sore throat, constipation, stomach ulcers, skin disorders, and many other conditions, but there is no good scientific evidence to support these uses.

Is it safe?
Slippery elm supplements seem to be safe for most adults. It can cause allergic reactions in sensitive people. Slippery elm ointment on the skin can sometimes cause a rash.

Sodium Bicarbonate (see Exercise and Athletic Performance)
Sodium bicarbonate, commonly known as baking soda or bicarbonate of soda, is a chemical compound with the formula $NaHCO_3$. It is a salt composed of a sodium cation and a bicarbonate anion. Sodium bicarbonate is a white solid that is crystalline, but often appears as a fine powder.

Does it work?
Sodium bicarbonate is an antacid used to relieve heartburn and acid indigestion. Your doctor also may prescribe sodium bicarbonate to make your blood or urine less acidic in certain conditions.

Is it safe?
When taken by mouth: Sodium bicarbonate is likely safe when used appropriately, short-term. Over-the-counter antacid products containing sodium bicarbonate are considered safe and effective by the US FDA. Taking sodium bicarbonate in very high doses is possibly unsafe.

Siberian Ginseng (ciwujia)
Eleutherococcus senticosus is a species of small, woody shrub in the family Araliaceae native to Northeastern Asia. It may be colloquially called devil's bush, Siberian ginseng,

eleuthero, ciwujia, Devil's shrub, shigoka, touch-me-not, wild pepper, or kan jang.

Does it work?

Quality of life. Some research shows that Siberian ginseng significantly improves sociability and sense of well-being in people over 65 years of age after 4 weeks of treatment. But the effects seem to disappear after 8 weeks. Alzheimer's disease.

Is it safe?

Siberian ginseng is likely safe for most adults when taken by mouth, short-term. While side effects are rare, some people can have drowsiness, changes in heart rhythm, sadness, anxiety, muscle spasms, and other side effects. In high doses, increased blood pressure might occur.

Soy

Soy (Glycine max) comes from soybeans. The beans are a legume that come from China. They can be processed into soy protein, soy milk, or soy fiber. Soy contains isoflavones which are changed in the body to phytoestrogens. Phytoestrogen molecules are similar in chemical structure to the hormone estrogen.

Does it work?

Soy is used for high cholesterol, high blood pressure, heart disease, diabetes, symptoms of menopause, and premenstrual syndrome (PMS). It is also used for many other conditions, but there is no good scientific evidence to support many of these uses.

Is it safe?

Except for people with soy allergies, soy is considered to be a safe food. In research studies, soy protein supplements and soy extracts rich in isoflavones have been used safely on a short-term basis; the safety of long-term use is uncertain.

Spearmint

Spearmint, or Mentha spicata is a pleasant-smelling species of mint found in health-food products, toothpastes, mouthwashes, and cosmetics. It is often used in medicine for its claimed therapeutic properties. Spearmint contains vitamins, antioxidants, and vital nutrients.

Does it work?
The Bottom Line. Spearmint is a delicious, minty herb that may have beneficial effects on your health. It's high in antioxidants and other beneficial plant compounds that may help balance hormones, lower blood sugar and improve digestion. It may even reduce stress and improve memory.

Is it safe?
When taken by mouth: Spearmint and spearmint oil are LIKELY SAFE when eaten in amounts commonly found in food. Spearmint is POSSIBLY SAFE when taken by mouth as a medicine, short-term. Side effects are very uncommon. Some people might have an allergic reaction to spearmint.

St. John's Wort
Hypericum perforatum, known as perforate St John's-wort, is a flowering plant in the family Hypericaceae and the type species of the genus Hypericum.

Does it work?
Several studies support the therapeutic benefit of St. John's wort in treating mild to moderate depression. In fact, some research has shown the supplement to be as effective as several prescription antidepressants. It's unclear whether it's beneficial in the treatment of severe depression.

Is it safe?
When taken orally for up to 12 weeks in appropriate doses, St. John's wort is generally considered safe. However, it may cause: Agitation and anxiety.

T

Tart or Sour Cherry (see Exercise and Athletic Performance)
Sour cherry (Prunus cerasus), also commonly called tart cherry, is a fruit. The Montmorency sour cherry is the most popular type grown in the U.S. Sour cherry fruit contains chemicals that might reduce swelling and act as antioxidants.

Does it work?
Research shows that the antioxidants in tart cherry juice can reduce pain and inflammation from osteoarthritis (OA). A

2012 study showed that drinking cherry juice twice a day for 21 days reduced the pain felt by people with OA. Blood tests also showed that they experienced significantly less inflammation.

Is it safe?

Could help you sleep better. Tart cherry juice may be a safe and effective way to treat insomnia and increase the amount of sleep you get each night. That's because tart cherries are naturally rich in melatonin, a hormone responsible for sleepiness.

Theanine

Theanine, also known as L-γ-glutamylethylamide and N^5-ethyl-L-glutamine, is an amino acid analogue of the proteinogenic amino acids L-glutamate and L-glutamine and is found primarily in particular plant and fungal species.

Does it work?

Theanine is found to be relaxing, but not sedating agent, and has been found to help process stress and to improve attention. It has also been found to aid in sleep quality. When combined with caffeine–like green or black tea–theanine is found to effectively cause improved cognition and attention.

Is it safe?

When taken by mouth: L-theanine is possibly safe when used short-term. Doses of up to 900 mg daily have been safely used for 8 weeks. It isn't clear if L-theanine is safe to use for longer periods of time. It might cause mild side effects, such as headache or sleepiness.

Tea

Tea is an aromatic beverage prepared by pouring hot or boiling water over cured or fresh leaves of Camellia sinensis, an evergreen shrub native to China and other East Asian countries. After water, it is the most widely consumed drink in the world.

Does it work?

Numerous studies have shown that a variety of teas may boost your immune system, fight off inflammation, and even ward off cancer and heart disease. While some brews provide more health advantages than others, there's plenty of evidence that regularly drinking tea can have a lasting impact on your wellness.

Is it safe?
Though moderate intake is healthy for most people, drinking too much could lead to negative side effects, such as anxiety, headaches, digestive issues, and disrupted sleep patterns. Most people can drink 3–4 cups (710–950 ml) of tea daily without adverse effects, but some may experience side effects at lower doses.

Thiamin
Thiamin (or thiamine) is one of the water-soluble B vitamins. It is also known as vitamin B1. Thiamin is naturally present in some foods, added to some food products, and available as a dietary supplement.

Does it work?
Thiamin (vitamin B1) helps the body's cells change carbohydrates into energy. The main role of carbohydrates is to provide energy for the body, especially the brain and nervous system. Thiamin also plays a role in muscle contraction and conduction of nerve signals.

Is it safe?
When used as an oral supplement in appropriate doses, thiamin is likely safe. Rarely, it can cause a skin reaction.

Tart or Sour Cherry
Sour cherries are also called "tart" cherries because even fruit needs marketing.

Does it work?
Research shows that the antioxidants in tart cherry juice can reduce pain and inflammation from osteoarthritis (OA). A 2012 study showed that drinking cherry juice twice a day for 21 days reduced the pain felt by people with OA. Blood tests also showed that they experienced significantly less inflammation.

Is it safe?
Tart cherry juice also contains quercetin, a plant compound that may interact with certain medications, particularly blood

thinners. Individuals on medications should consult a doctor before adding large amounts of tart cherry juice to their diet. Summary: Tart cherry juice is considered safe for most people.

Trametes versicolor or Coriolus versicolor
Trametes versicolor also known as Coriolus versicolor and Polyporus versicolor is a common polypore mushroom found throughout the world. Meaning 'of several colors', versicolor reliably describes this fungus that displays a variety of colors.

Does it work?
Studies during the 1990s established that C. versicolor polysaccharides such as PSK could inhibit hepatic carcinogenesis in rats induced by 3'-methyl-4-dimethylaminoazobenzene. The direct effect of PSK on gene expression profile in cancer cells was also established back in the 1980s.

Is it safe?
Turkey tail mushroom is considered safe, with few side effects reported in research studies. Some people may experience digestive symptoms like gas, bloating and dark stools when taking turkey tail mushroom.

Thunder God Vine
Tripterygium wilfordii, or léi gōng téng, sometimes called thunder god vine but more properly translated thunder duke vine, is a vine used in traditional Chinese medicine.

Does it work?
Preliminary research suggests that oral or topical thunder god vine might be beneficial for rheumatoid arthritis symptoms. Some studies have suggested that thunder god vine plus standard medical treatment may be more effective than standard treatment alone for symptoms such as joint swelling and tenderness.

Is it safe?
Thunder god vine may have side effects, including digestive problems, abnormal heart rates, high blood pressure, less blood cell production, kidney problems, decreased bone mineral content (with long-term use), infertility, menstrual cycle changes, rashes, diarrhea, headache, and hair loss.

Tribulus

Tribulus (Tribulus terrestris) is a plant that produces fruit covered with spines. It is traditionally known as an aphrodisiac in various cultures.

Does it work?

Use tribulus for sexual disorders, infertility, chest pain, enlarged prostate, and many other conditions, but there is no good scientific evidence to support most of these uses.

Is it safe?

When taken by mouth: Tribulus is possibly safe for most people when taken at doses of 750-1500 mg daily for up to 90 days. Side effects are usually mild and uncommon, but might include stomach pain, cramping, and diarrhea.

Turmeric

Turmeric is a flowering plant, Curcuma longa, of the ginger family, Zingiberaceae, the rhizomes of which are used in cooking.

Does it work?

Turmeric — and especially its most active compound, curcumin — have many scientifically proven health benefits, such as the potential to improve heart health and prevent against Alzheimer's and cancer. It's a potent anti-inflammatory and antioxidant. It may also help improve symptoms of depression and arthritis.

Is it safe?

Turmeric is generally safe. It can cause nausea and diarrhea, especially in high doses or after long-term use. It might also pose a risk of ulcers in high doses. As a topical treatment, it can cause skin irritation.

V

Valerian

Valerian is a perennial flowering plant native to Europe and Asia. In the summer when the mature plant may have a height of 1.5 metres, it bears sweetly scented pink or white flowers that attract many fly species, especially hoverflies of the genus Eristalis.

Does it work?

Some studies show that it helps people fall asleep faster and feel that they have a better quality of sleep. One of the best designed studies found that valerian was no more effective than placebo for 14 days, but by 28 days valerian greatly improved sleep for those who were taking it.

Is it safe?

Research suggests that valerian is generally safe for short-term use by most adults. It has been used with apparent safety in studies lasting up to 28 days. The safety of long-term use of valerian is unknown. Little is known about whether it's safe to use valerian during pregnancy or while breastfeeding.

Vanadium

Vanadium is a rare, hard, ductile gray-white element found combined in certain minerals and used mainly to produce certain alloys. Vanadium resists corrosion due to a protective film of oxide on the surface. Common oxidation states of vanadium include +2, +3, +4 and +5.

Does it work?

A silvery metal that resists corrosion. About 80% of the vanadium produced is used as a steel additive. Vanadium-steel alloys are very tough and are used for armour plate, axles, tools, piston rods and crankshafts. Less than 1% of vanadium, and as little chromium, makes steel shock resistant and vibration resistant.

Is it safe?

When taken by mouth: Vanadium is likely safe in adults if taken by mouth in amounts less than 1.8 mg per day. Vanadium is possibly safe when taken by mouth in higher amounts. At higher doses, vanadium often causes unwanted side effects including stomach discomfort, diarrhea, nausea, and gas.

Valine (see Exercise and Athletic Performance)

Valine is a branched-chain essential amino acid that has stimulant activity. It promotes muscle growth and tissue repair. It is a precursor in the penicillin biosynthetic pathway.

Does it work?

Valine helps stimulate muscle growth and regeneration and is involved in energy production. Threonine. This is a principal part of structural proteins, such as collagen and elastin, which are important components of your skin and connective tissue. It also plays a role in fat metabolism and immune function.

Is it safe?
The FEEDAP Panel concludes that the additive l-valine produced by C. glutamicum KCCM 11201P is safe for all animal species when supplemented in appropriate amounts to the diet. No risks are expected for the consumer from the use of l-valine produced by C. glutamicum KCCM 11201P as a feed additive.

Vinpocetine
Vinpocetine is a man-made chemical similar to a substance found in the periwinkle plant (Vinca minor). In Europe, it's sold as a drug called Cavinton. Vinpocetine might increase blood flow to the brain and protect brain cells (neurons) against injury.

Does it work?
Vinpocetine might increase blood flow to the brain and protect brain cells (neurons) against injury. People use vinpocetine for memory, dementia, stroke, hearing loss, and many other conditions, but there is no good scientific evidence to support most of these uses.

Is it safe?
When taken by mouth: Vinpocetine is possibly safe for most people when used appropriately for up to one year. It can cause some side effects including anxiety, stomach discomfort, sleep problems, headache, dizziness, and flushing of the face.

Vitamin A
Vitamin A is a fat-soluble vitamin and an essential nutrient for humans. It is a group of organic compounds that includes retinol, retinal (also known as retinaldehyde), retinoic acid, and several provitamin A carotenoids (most notably beta-carotene (β-carotene). Vitamin A has multiple functions: it is essential for embryo development and growth, for maintenance of the immune system, and for vision, where it combines with the

protein opsin to form rhodopsin – the light-absorbing molecule necessary for both low-light (scotopic vision) and color vision.

Does it work?

Vitamin A helps form and maintain healthy teeth, skeletal and soft tissue, mucus membranes, and skin. It is also known as retinol because it produces the pigments in the retina of the eye. Vitamin A promotes good eyesight, especially in low light. It also has a role in healthy pregnancy and breastfeeding.

Is it safe?

Since too much vitamin A can be harmful, consult with your doctor before taking vitamin A supplements. Vitamin A toxicity may cause symptoms, such as liver damage, vision disturbances, nausea and even death. High-dose vitamin A supplements should be avoided unless prescribed by your doctor.

Vitamin D

Your body needs vitamin D for good health and strong bones. People who are obese tend to have lower levels of vitamin D, but there is no known reason why taking vitamin D would help people lose weight.

Does it work?

Vitamin D doesn't help you lose weight.

Is it safe?

Vitamin D from foods and dietary supplements is safe at the recommended amounts of 600–800 IU a day for adults. Too much vitamin D (more than 4,000 IU a day) can be toxic and cause nausea, vomiting, poor appetite, constipation, weakness, and irregular heartbeat.

W

Weight Loss

Weight loss is a decrease in body weight resulting from either voluntary (diet, exercise) or involuntary (illness) circumstances. Most instances of weight loss arise due to the loss of body fat, but in cases of extreme or severe weight loss, protein and other substances in the body can also be depleted.

Whey protein

Whey is the liquid remaining after milk has been curdled and strained. It is a byproduct of the manufacturing of cheese or casein and has several commercial uses. Sweet whey is a byproduct resulting from the manufacture of rennet types of hard cheese, like cheddar or Swiss cheese.

Does it work?

Taking whey protein is a great way to increase your protein intake, which should have major benefits for weight loss. Studies have shown that replacing other sources of calories with whey protein, combined with weight lifting, can cause weight loss of about 8 pounds (3.5 kg) while increasing lean muscle mass.

Is it safe?

When taken in appropriate amounts, whey protein appears to be safe. Some research suggests that whey protein might cause gastrointestinal discomfort. However, there's limited data on the possible side effects of high protein intake from a combination of food and supplements.

White kidney bean (see Weight Loss)

White kidney bean or bean pod (also called Phaseolus vulgaris) is a legume grown around the world. An extract of this bean is claimed to block the absorption of carbohydrates and suppress your appetite.

Does it work?

Phaseolus vulgaris extract might help you lose a small amount of weight and body fat.

Is it safe?

Phaseolus vulgaris seems to be safe (at up to 3,000 mg a day for 12 weeks). But it might cause headaches, soft stools, flatulence, and constipation.

Wormwood

Wormwood (Artemisia absinthium) is an herb used in the alcoholic drinks vermouth and absinthe. Its oil contains the chemical thujone, which may be poisonous. The thujone in wormwood oil excites the central nervous system and can cause seizures and other adverse effects.

Does it work?

People use wormwood for digestion problems, Crohn disease, a kidney disorder called IgA nephropathy, osteoarthritis, and many other conditions, but there is no good scientific evidence to support these uses. There is also no good evidence to support using wormwood for COVID-19.

Is it safe?
Thujone-free wormwood is possibly safe when used as medicine, short-term. But wormwood that contains thujone is possibly unsafe. Thujone can cause seizures, kidney failure, vomiting, and other serious side effects. When applied to the skin: Wormwood extract is possibly safe as an ointment.Moringa Leaf Powder

Wild yam
Dioscorea villosa is a species of twining tuberous vine which is native to eastern North America. It is commonly known as wild yam, colic root, rheumatism root, devil's bones, and fourleaf yam. It is common and widespread in a range stretching from Texas and Florida north to Minnesota, Ontario and Massachusetts.

Does it work?
There might be other chemicals in wild yam that act like estrogen in the body. People most commonly use wild yam as a "natural alterative" to estrogen therapy for symptoms of menopause, infertility, menstrual problems, and many other conditions, but there is no good scientific evidence to support any of these uses.

Is it safe?
When taken by mouth: Wild yam is possibly safe when used for up to 12 weeks. It's usually well tolerated, but taking large amounts might cause vomiting, upset stomach, and headache. When applied to the skin: Wild yam is possibly safe when applied to the skin.

Willow bark
Willow bark comes from several varieties of willow tree, including white (Salix alba or European), black (Salix nigra or pussy), crack, and purple willow.

Does it work?

Limited evidence suggests that willow bark may have a moderate effect in treating pain caused by osteoarthritis and rheumatoid arthritis. In the single study testing it against a non-steroidal anti-inflammatory drug (NSAID) for osteoarthritis, it wasn't as effective for pain relief.

Is it safe?
When taken by mouth: Willow bark is possibly safe when used for up to 12 weeks. It might cause diarrhea, heartburn, and vomiting in some people. It can also cause itching, rash, and allergic reactions, particularly in people who are allergic to aspirin.

Y

Yerba mate
Yerba mate or yerba-maté is a plant species of the holly genus Ilex native to South America. It was named by the French botanist Augustin Saint-Hilaire. The indigenous Guaraní and some Tupí communities first cultivated and used yerba mate prior to European colonization of the Americas.

Does it work?
In the U.S., yerba mate is widely available in health food stores and online. People who recommend yerba mate say that it can relieve fatigue, aid in weight loss, ease depression, and help treat headaches and various other conditions. There's limited evidence that yerba mate may help with some of these conditions.

Is it safe?
Yerba mate isn't likely to pose a risk for healthy adults who occasionally drink it. However, some studies indicate that people who drink large amounts of yerba mate over long periods may be at increased risk of some types of cancer, such as cancer of the mouth, throat and lungs.

Yohimbe
Yohimbe is a West African tree. Yohimbe, which contains a compound called yohimbine, is an ingredient found in some dietary supplements claiming to increase weight loss, improve libido, increase muscle mass, or treat male sexual dysfunction.

Does it work?
Yohimbe doesn't help you lose weight.

Is it safe?
Yohimbe might not be safe (especially at yohimbine doses of 20 mg or higher). Use it only with guidance from your healthcare provider because the side effects can be severe. Yohimbe can cause headaches, high blood pressure, anxiety, agitation, rapid heartbeat, heart attack, heart failure, and death.

Z

Zinc
Zinc is a chemical element with the symbol Zn and atomic number 30. Zinc is a slightly brittle metal at room temperature and has a silvery-greyish appearance when oxidation is removed. It is the first element in group 12 of the periodic table.

Does it work?
Zinc may work by preventing the rhinovirus from multiplying. It may also stop the rhinovirus from lodging in the mucous membranes of the throat and nose. Zinc may be more effective when taken in lozenge or syrup form, which allows the substance to stay in the throat and come in contact with the rhinovirus.

Is it safe?
Taking very high doses of zinc is likely unsafe and might cause stomach pain, vomiting, and many other problems. Single doses of 10-30 grams of zinc can be fatal. When applied to the skin: Zinc is likely safe. Using zinc on broken skin may cause burning, stinging, itching, and tingling.

About the Author

Dr. Ernesto Martinez suffered a near-fatal assault that changed the direction of his life. The experience helped him acquire a greater moral understanding and develop greater empathy for others.

Martinez is a Naturopathic Doctor, Occupational Therapist, and Investor. He also enjoys writing, publishing, traveling, blogging AttaBoyCowboy.com, and running his YouTube channel AttaBoyCowboy.

So be sure to check out his fun books, blog, and YouTube channel.

Martinez's work as a Naturopathic Doctor specializes in anti-aging medicine and complementary cancer therapies. He focuses on a whole-body treatment approach utilizing safe natural methods, while simultaneously restoring the body's natural ability to heal.

His work as an Occupational Therapist has allowed him to help people across the lifespan to do things they want and need to do to live their life to the fullest. His strong desire to mentor and help others has led him to teach, share, and help them live better lives.

As an Investor, Martinez has focused his training and business acumen on real estate. With a family history of real estate investing and extensive academic training, he has developed innovative strategies for building wealth from nothing.

In addition to his medical practice and three decades of investing experience, Martinez is making his impact on the writing and media field. Through his books, blog, and YouTube channel, he is reaching a broad spectrum of people and teaching them how to live healthier and wealthier lives.

Martinez has taught extension courses for the University of San Diego in topics ranging from nutrition and general health to leadership and business. He holds five associate degrees from Cerritos College, a bachelor's degree from the University of Southern California (USC), an MBA in economics and marketing, and a master's degree in healthcare management (MHCM) from California State University Los Angeles (CSULA), a doctoral degree from Clayton College, and over ten other degrees and advanced certifications in areas including lifestyle redesign and nutrition, alternative nutrition, assistive technology, sensory integration, neuro-developmental treatment, physical agent modalities, lymphedema treatment, and property management. He studied over fifteen years working his entire academic career and for several years attending two graduate schools on two separate campuses at the same time.

He is a huge fan of all sports, reading, and being on the road traveling!

As an entrepreneur, Ernesto is usually problem-solving business issues, writing, and learning to be a better person. He enjoys spending time with his family and friends.

By far one of his favorite activities is practicing his Random Acts of Kindness, where he tries to do three acts of kindness for strangers a day.

Ernesto Martinez

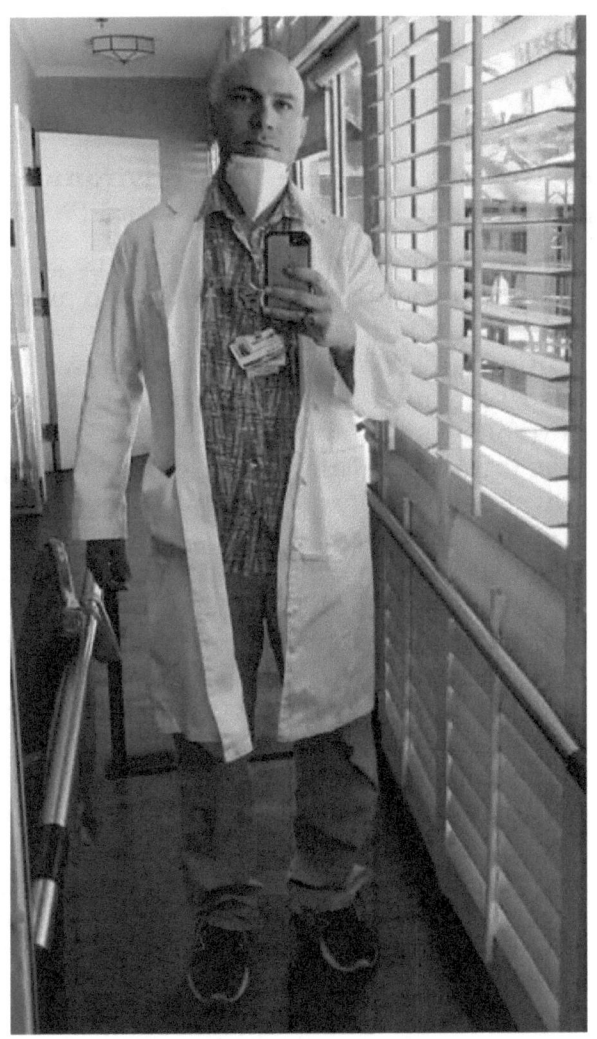

Bonus

Top Ten Ways to Decrease Your Environmental Impact During Travel per World Wildlife Fund (WWF)

1. Go on holiday during the off-peak period to prevent overstraining resources; you'll also avoid the crowds.
2. Find out about places before you visit. You may be visiting an environmentally sensitive area, in which case you must take extra care to stay on footpaths and follow signs.
3. Don't travel by air if you can avoid it, because air travel uses up large amounts of jet fuel that releases greenhouse gases.
4. Dispose of any rubbish responsibly; it can be hazardous to wildlife.
5. Use public transportation, cycle or walk instead of using a car.
6. Use facilities and trips run by local people whenever possible.
7. Don't be tempted to touch wildlife and disturb habitats whether on land, at the coast, or under water.
8. Be careful what you choose to bring home as a holiday souvenir. Many species from coral and conch shells to elephants and alligators are endangered because they are killed for curios or souvenirs.
9. Don't dump chemicals into the environment; it can be very dangerous for wildlife.
10. Boats and jet-skis create noise and chemical pollution that is very disturbing to wildlife; don't keep the engine running unnecessarily

Top Ten Ways to Decrease Your Environmental Impact after Travel per WWF

1. Completely turn off equipment like televisions and stereos when you're not using them.

2. Choose energy-efficient appliances and light bulbs.
3. Save water: some simple steps can go a long way in saving water, like turning off the tap when you are brushing your teeth or shaving. Try to collect the water used to wash vegetables and salad to water your houseplants.
4. Lower your shades or close your curtains on hot days, to keep the house fresh and reduce the use of electric fans or air-conditioning.
5. Let clothes dry naturally.
6. Keep lids on pans when cooking to conserve energy.
7. Use rechargeable batteries.
8. Call your local government to see if they have a disposal location for used batteries, glass, plastics, paper, or other wastes.
9. Don't use "throwaway" products like paper plates and napkins or plastic knives, forks, and cups.
10. Send electronic greetings over email instead of paper cards.

Top Ten Ways to Decrease Your Environmental Impact in the Garden per WWF

1. Collect rainwater to water your garden.
2. Water the garden early in the morning or late in the evening. Water loss is reduced due to evaporation. Don't over-water the garden. Water only until the soil becomes moist, not soggy.
3. Explore water-efficient irrigation systems. Sprinkler irrigation and drip irrigation can be adapted to garden situations.
4. Make your garden lively, plant trees, and shrubs that will attract birds. You can also put up bird nest boxes with food.
5. Put waste to work in your garden, sweep the fallen leaves and flowers into flowerbeds, or under shrubs. Increasing soil fertility and also reduce the need for frequent watering.
6. If you have little space in your garden, you could make a compost pit to turn organic waste from the kitchen and garden to soil-enriching manure.

7. Plant local species of trees, flowers, and vegetables.
8. Don't use chemicals in the garden, as they will eventually end up in the water systems and can upset the delicate balance of life cycles.
9. Organic and environmentally friendly fertilizers and pesticides are available - organic gardening reduces pollution and is better for wildlife.
10. Buy fruit and vegetables that are in season to help reduce enormous transport costs resulting from importing products and, where possible, choose locally produced food.

Top Ten Ways to Reduce, Reuse, and Recycle per WWF

1. Use email to stay in touch, including cards, rather than faxing or writing.
2. Share magazines with friends and pass them on to the doctor, dentist, or local hospital for their waiting rooms.
3. Use recyclable paper to make invitation cards, envelopes, letter pads, etc. if you can.
4. Use washable nappies instead of disposables, if you can.
5. Recycle as much as you can.
6. Give unwanted clothes, toys, and books to charities and orphanages.
7. Store food and other products in containers rather than foil and plastic wrap.
8. When buying fish, look out for a variety of non-endangered species, and buy local fish if possible.
9. Bring your bags to the grocery and refuse plastic bags that create so much waste.
10. Look for products that have less packaging.

Top Ten Ways to Reduce Your Environmental Impact at Work per WWF

1. Always use both sides of a sheet of paper.

2. Use printers that can print on both sides of the paper; try to look into this option when replacing old printers.
3. Use the back of a draft or unwanted printout instead of notebooks. Even with a double-sided printer, there is likely to be plenty of spare paper to use!
4. Always ask for and buy recycled paper if you can, for your business stationery, and to use it in your printers.
5. Switch off computer monitors, printers, and other equipment at the end of each day. Always turn off your office light and computer monitor when you go out for lunch or to a meeting.
6. Look for power-saving alternatives like LED light bulbs, motion-sensing to control the lighting, LED computer monitors, etc. Prioritize buying or replacing equipment and appliances with their higher Energy Rating alternatives.
7. Contact your energy provider and what they offer in the way of green energy alternatives. You could install solar panels to reduce reliance on energy providers if they're slow on the green energy uptake.
8. Carpool. Ask your workmates that live nearby if they'd be happy to share rides with you.
9. Be smarter with your company vehicles. When reviewing your fleet, spend some time researching more efficient cars.
10. Clean and maintain equipment regularly to extend their useful life and avoid having to replace them. Just like getting your vehicle serviced regularly, your floors, kitchens, equipment, and bathrooms all need regular attention to protect their form and function.

Made in United States
Troutdale, OR
11/28/2023

14980555R00156